Introduction

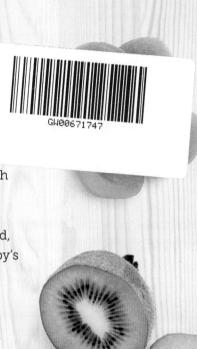

Thank you for choosing to read **Carbs & Cals GESTATIONAL DIAF** This book is a support guide for people who have been diagnosed with gestational diabetes, and those who are at risk of developing it. If this is you, you may be feeling overwhelmed, anxious or concerned about your baby's health and how your pregnancy will continue. A diagnosis of gestational diabetes can potentially overshadow the joy and excitement of pregnancy.

View it from a different angle and it can be a unique opportunity for you to focus on your self-care, and in doing so, ensure your baby gets the best start in life. The diagnosis does demand greater focus on your diet and lifestyle; for example, working out how to fit in more physical activity and a crash course in nutrition (learning how different foods affect your blood glucose levels), not to mention making more time for hospital appointments. However, this also gives you the chance to take a little more time for yourself, which is something that today's fast-paced lifestyles rarely allow.

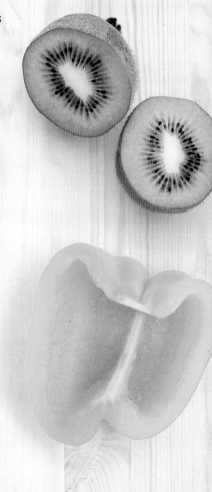

When you are newly diagnosed, question marks start to surround every day activities such as socialising, physical activity, eating and drinking. The dietary approach to managing gestational diabetes emphasises nutrient-rich foods that provide your baby with all the critical nutrients for growth, whilst minimising blood glucose spikes. The good news is that managed well, with good blood glucose control, your risk of complications can be the same as for a woman who doesn't have diabetes.

This book will show you what you can eat, offering inspiration about new foods and how they can be included in your diet. It will also help you make healthy changes to your nutrition and physical activity habits that can last a lifetime, benefiting you, your family and those closest to you.

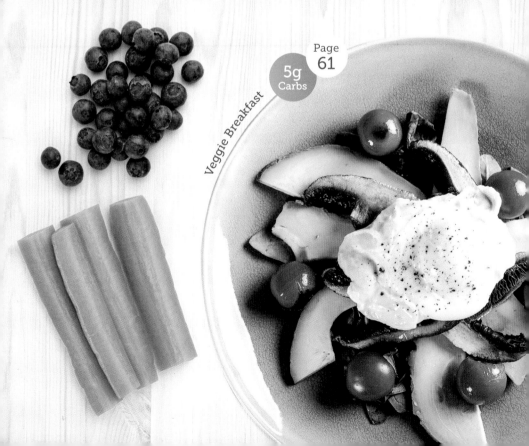

Page
61

5g
Carbs

Veggie Breakfast

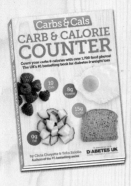

CARB & CALORIE COUNTER

★ Over 1,700 food & drink photos

★ A visual way to count carbs, calories, protein, fat, fibre and 5-a-day fruit & veg

★ The essential resource for diabetes, portion control & healthy eating

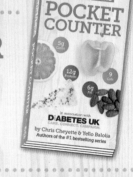

POCKET COUNTER

★ Over 750 food & drink photos

★ Great accompaniment to the **CARB & CALORIE COUNTER**

★ Perfect when out and about!

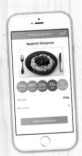 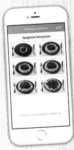

MOBILE APP

Available for iPhone & Android

★ Over 3,500 photos, including branded foods

★ Perfect for weight loss, portion control & diabetes

★ The ultimate portable calorie counter!

PLUS...
FREE HEALTH RESOURCES

FREE!

★ Register for FREE access to 50 PDF resources

★ www.carbsandcals.com/register

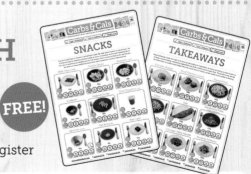

Visit www.carbsandcals.com

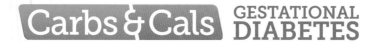

Carbs & Cals GESTATIONAL DIABETES

1ST EDITION

First published in Great Britain in 2018
by Chello Publishing Limited
Registered Company Number 7237986
www.chellopublishing.co.uk | info@chellopublishing.co.uk

Copyright © Chello Publishing Limited 2018

With special thanks to Fran Turner, George Malache, Gian Mizzi, Gordon Caruana, Justine Rose, Maxine Gregory, Mike Rogers, Simon Callaghan, Tom Maund, Victoria Francis and Yoshi Balolia.

Nutritional information for the African-Caribbean dishes was used with permission from the World Food Study, King's College London. We are grateful to Dr Louise Goff and Annemarie Knight for providing access to the World Food Study data, and to Amanda Moore for undertaking nutritional composition analysis.

All rights reserved. No part of this work may be reproduced or utilised in any form or by any means, electronic or mechanical, including photocopying, recording, or by any information storage and retrieval system, without the prior written permission of the publishers and authors.

The information contained in this book is not a substitute for medical or other professional guidance. Please consult your GP before making any alterations to medications or changing medical treatment. Although all reasonable care has been taken in the writing of this book, the authors and publisher are not responsible for any specific health needs; they do not accept any legal responsibility or liability for any personal injury or other consequences, damage or loss arising from any use of information and advice contained within this book.

The authors have asserted their moral rights.

ISBN: 978-1-908261-22-9 Printed in Malta 1217

Authors	Chris Cheyette BSc (Hons) MSc RD Yello Balolia BA (Hons)
Recipes by	Chris Cheyette BSc (Hons) MSc RD Victoria Francis BSc (Hons) RD
Photography	Simon Callaghan & Francesca Turner
Design Concept	George F Malache
Graphic Design	Maxine Gregory BA (Hons)
Additional Layout	Yello Balolia BA (Hons)
Introduction Text	Victoria Francis BSc (Hons) RD
Assistant Dietitian	Monika Jakiel-Rusin BSc (Hons) MSc RD

For more information, please visit:

www.carbsandcals.com

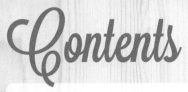Contents

Foreword 4
Introduction 5
   What you can eat to manage your diabetes 12
   How to use this book 30
   What next? 38
Meal Plans 40
Recipes 54
   Breakfasts 54
   Curries 74
   General Meals 82
   Salads 108
   Soups & Stews 118
   Snacks 134
Individual Foods 144
   Bread 144
   Cereals 146
   Cheese 147
   Drinks 150
   Eggs & Vegetarian 151
   Fish 152
   Fruit 156
   Herbs 168
   Meat 169
   Milk 172
   Nuts & Seeds 174
   Rice, Pasta & Grains 178
   Spreads & Sauces 182
   Vegetables 191
   Other 214
Index 216
   Recipe Index 216
   Ingredient Index 217
About the Authors / Awards 222

Foreword

We know there's a lot to think about when you're having a baby, and now that you've been diagnosed with gestational diabetes, you probably have a lot of questions. The good news is that by managing gestational diabetes properly, you can have a healthy pregnancy and birth.

Carbs & Cals: Gestational Diabetes is more than just a recipe book. From carbohydrate counting to expert advice, it offers simple, evidence-based information so you can understand more about your diabetes and make healthier choices at meal times.

Use this essential resource alongside advice from your healthcare professional to build an approach that works for you, making sure you have the right knowledge at the right time to have a healthy and enjoyable pregnancy.

Chris Askew
Chief Executive Officer, Diabetes UK

DiABETES UK
KNOW DIABETES. FIGHT DIABETES.

www.diabetes.org.uk

What is gestational diabetes?

Diabetes is a condition in which the body can't control the amount of glucose (sugar) in the blood. Gestational diabetes is a type of diabetes that affects pregnant women, commonly in their second or third trimester. 'Gestational' simply means 'relating to pregnancy'. Many people are surprised to learn that gestational diabetes is fairly common, affecting 1 in 7 pregnancies globally. Research shows that about 16% (or 1 in 6) of pregnant women in the UK have gestational diabetes.

Glucose is needed by the body to provide energy, and levels of glucose are controlled by the hormone insulin. After eating a meal containing carbohydrate, blood glucose levels rise. This causes insulin to be produced, which allows glucose to be used up by cells or stored for later use. When you are pregnant, your body produces high levels of hormones to support the growth of your baby. Some of these hormones stop insulin working as well as it normally does. Usually, the body responds by increasing the amount of insulin it produces. However, some women do not produce enough of this extra insulin, or the insulin produced is not used by the body (known as 'insulin resistance'). This leads to high glucose levels in the blood and a diagnosis of gestational diabetes.

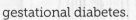

Prawn & Kale Stir-fry

20g Carbs

Page 88

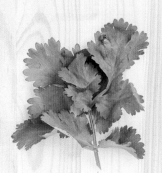

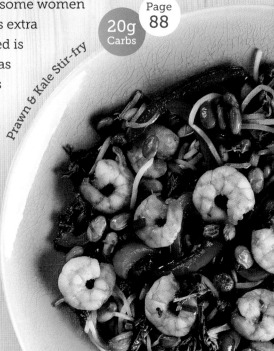

What does it mean for me and my baby?

Gestational diabetes is a serious medical condition that, if left untreated, can have consequences for you and your baby. The more glucose there is in your blood, the more your baby will be exposed to. This extra glucose puts your baby at risk of growing too large, which may lead to a more difficult delivery for both you and your baby. If not managed properly, persistent high blood glucose levels carry other risk factors including prematurity, your baby having low blood glucose levels, and you and your baby having a higher risk of being overweight or developing type 2 diabetes in later life.

However, gestational diabetes can be treated successfully, and does not have to affect the health of your baby. It will probably mean a change to your expected pregnancy experience and there are likely to be changes to your birthing plan. As already stated, there will be more trips to your healthcare team (look at this as a chance to check-in with your baby more, thanks to regular scans), testing of your blood glucose levels at home and a greater focus on your diet, which is also likely to see changes. These are all important to ensure you and your baby are kept healthy throughout your pregnancy.

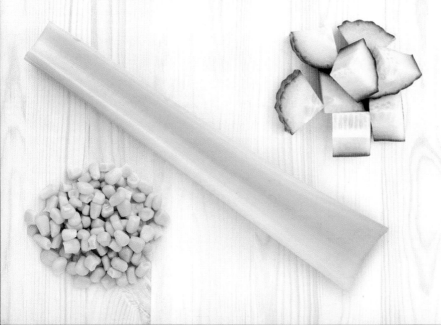

What treatment is available?

The primary treatment for gestational diabetes is diet and physical activity, as both have a direct impact on blood glucose levels. You are now most probably aware that what you do and what you eat have a great impact on the health of you, your pregnancy and your baby. When diet and physical activity aren't enough to keep blood glucose levels within the normal range, you may need medication and/or insulin. For some women, medication may need to be started at diagnosis.

The choice of treatment depends on what will have the greatest impact on your blood glucose levels and what is tolerated by you. Metformin is a tablet used to help reduce the amount of glucose produced by the liver and make the insulin work more effectively. Evidence supports the use of metformin in pregnancy. It is taken with meals, or immediately after. In addition to metformin, insulin may be required. Injecting insulin ensures there is enough insulin in your body to control your blood glucose levels. Your healthcare team will advise on which type of insulin to use, how to inject it, dispose of needles and ensure your safety whilst using it. It is important to be aware that metformin and insulin are used in conjunction with diet and are not standalone treatments.

Page
93

26g
Carbs

Tuna & Roasted Veg

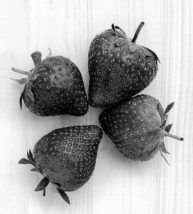

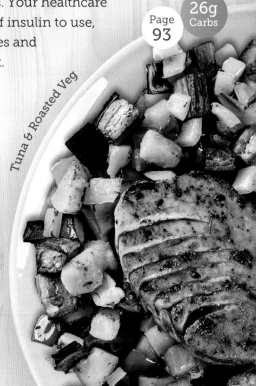

Physical activity recommendations

Don't put away your running shoes just yet! The proven benefits of physical activity during pregnancy include improved circulation, reduced likelihood of swelling (ankles, for example), improved sleep and reduced levels of stress and anxiety.

Physical activity also has a positive impact on blood glucose levels by increasing the amount of glucose used by muscles and helping to lower blood glucose levels. It also improves insulin sensitivity, which means that regular physical activity causes the body to use insulin more effectively.

The general advice for the adult population is 150 minutes of moderate intensity activity per week (e.g. 30 minutes, five times per week). Simple moderate intensity activities that are safe in pregnancy include walking, swimming, gardening, aqua aerobics and pregnancy pilates/yoga.

Simple tips for physical activity:

★ If you consider yourself physically inactive, introduce simple activities and build them up gradually.

★ Research has shown that physical activity after a meal is particularly useful in managing blood glucose levels. Try to do a 20-30 minute walk after eating.

★ Be careful not to overexert yourself. You should be able to comfortably hold a conversation while exercising.

★ If you have exercised regularly prior to your pregnancy then you can continue with the same higher intensity exercises you are used to.

★ If you are unsure about the level of exercise that is appropriate for you, check with your healthcare team.

Pregnancy with type 1 and type 2 diabetes

For women with type 1 and type 2 diabetes, the key to a healthy pregnancy is planning. Good blood glucose control, higher dose folic acid and a specific pre-conception medical review are all important factors prior to pregnancy. It is important to manage your blood glucose levels carefully from the start, as high blood glucose levels in the first trimester (when the baby's organs are forming) increase the risk of birth defects and miscarriage.

During pregnancy, your diabetes control will require more work. The target blood glucose values will be different, probably lower than usual, and you will be asked to do more frequent testing including pre and post-meal tests. Your diabetes medication plan will also change. For example, if you usually manage your diabetes with tablets, your healthcare team may switch to insulin straight away, as insulin resistance often decreases the effectiveness of oral diabetes medication. As pregnancy continues, your body's need for insulin will go up (this is especially true during the last three months of pregnancy).

Dietary advice remains the same for women irrespective of the type of diabetes. For women who are familiar with carb counting and insulin dose adjustment, this is encouraged during pregnancy. Although, your ratios are likely to increase as pregnancy continues.

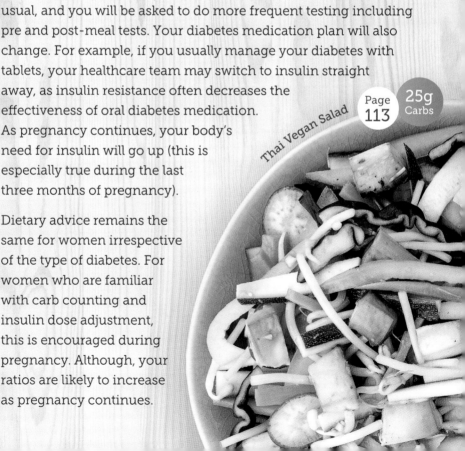

Thai Vegan Salad

Page 113

25g Carbs

What you can eat to manage your diabetes

When it comes to diet for gestational diabetes, the spotlight is on carbohydrate, as it is the main nutrient that causes a rise in blood glucose levels. During digestion, foods containing carbohydrate are broken down by the body into glucose - in other words, sugar. Glucose is the body's main source of energy (and the brain's preferred source of energy), so we still need some in the diet. But to control blood glucose levels, the focus needs to be on the **type** and **amount** of carbohydrate in the diet.

Types of carbohydrate

The two main types of carbs are starchy carbohydrates and sugars. Starchy carbs include bread, pasta, chapatis, potatoes, yam and cereals. Sugars can be categorised as natural sugars and added sugars (or 'free sugars'). Free sugars include those added to food by manufacturers, cooks or consumers (such as granulated sugar) and those naturally present in honey, syrups and unsweetened fruit juice.

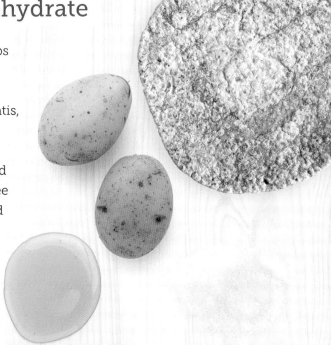

Glycaemic Index (GI)

Smart carbohydrate choices include those that don't cause your blood glucose levels to spike immediately after meals, because they are broken down more slowly. The rate at which carbohydrate is broken down depends on the type of carbohydrate consumed. This is known as the Glycaemic Index.

Food or drinks with a high GI are broken down quickly, causing a rapid rise in blood glucose levels.

Foods with a low GI are broken down slowly, giving a more gradual rise in blood glucose levels.

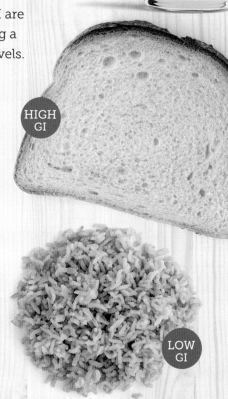

HIGH GI

HIGH GI

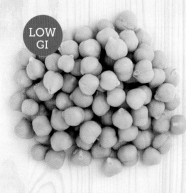

LOW GI

LOW GI

Choosing foods with a low GI will help you to manage your blood glucose levels and also keep you feeling full between meals. This is because low GI foods take longer for your body to digest, so glucose is released more slowly into your bloodstream.

Foods to avoid

These foods will cause a rapid rise in your blood glucose levels (high GI), so should be avoided or eaten in small quantities, and not on a regular basis:

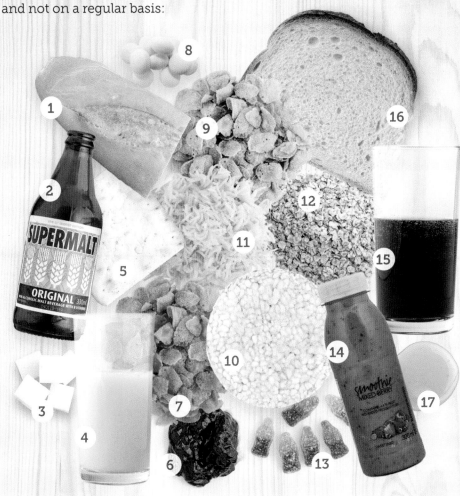

1. Baguette
2. Supermalt
3. Sugar
4. Orange juice
5. Cream crackers
6. Jam
7. Cornflakes
8. Mints
9. Sugar-coated cereal
10. Rice cakes
11. Long grain rice
12. Quick cook oats
13. Sweets
14. Smoothies (shop bought)
15. Fizzy drinks
16. White bread
17. Honey

Smart choices

The foods on this page are encouraged as they either contain little carbohydrate, or the carbohydrate they do contain is broken down slowly (low GI). These should be chosen as alternatives to high GI choices, where possible:

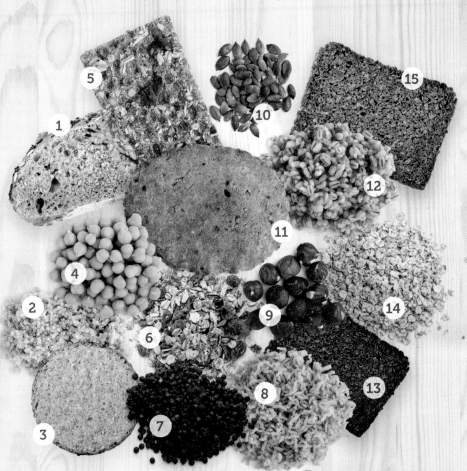

1. Sourdough bread	6. Nutty muesli	11. Wholemeal pitta bread
2. Quinoa	7. Lentils	12. Pearl barley
3. Oatcakes	8. Brown rice	13. Pumpernickel bread
4. Chickpeas	9. Nuts	14. Jumbo oats
5. Seeded crispbread	10. Seeds	15. Rye bread

Simple GI swaps

Carb choices which cause blood glucose to rise quickly (high GI):

Smart carb choices (low GI):

Bread:

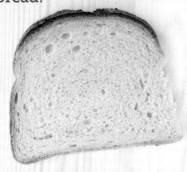

★ White bread
★ Wholemeal bread
★ Brown bread

Bread:

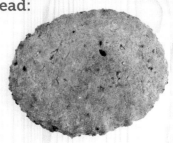

★ Multigrain / granary / seeded bread
★ Wholemeal pitta bread
★ Crispbread with seeds
★ Rye / pumpernickel bread

Rice & Grains:

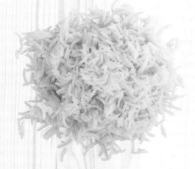

★ Instant rice
★ Long grain rice
★ Jasmine rice
★ Sticky rice

Rice & Grains:

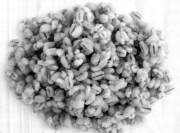

★ Basmati rice
★ Brown rice
★ Pearl barley
★ Buckwheat
★ Quinoa
★ Bulgur wheat

Carb choices which cause blood glucose to rise quickly (high GI):	Smart carb choices (low GI):

Cereal:

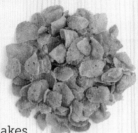

* ★ Corn Flakes
* ★ Rice Krispies
* ★ Quick cook porridge
* ★ Sugar and/or honey-covered cereals

Cereal:

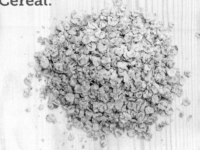

* ★ Jumbo oats
* ★ Nutty muesli

Fruit:

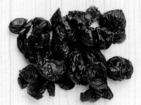

* ★ All fruit can be included in the diet but tropical & dried fruit can cause a big rise in your blood glucose levels

Fruit:

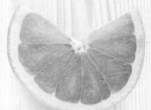

* ★ Berries
* ★ Cherries
* ★ Grapefruit

Potatoes:

* ★ Baked potato
* ★ Mashed potato
* ★ Boiled potato (no skin)

Potatoes:

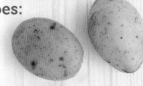

* ★ Sweet potato
* ★ New potatoes (boiled, with skin)

Amount of carbohydrate

As the saying goes: 'You can have too much of a good thing'. It is agreed by all healthcare professionals that the amount of carbohydrate in a meal is a good predictor of how high blood glucose levels will rise. In other words, the larger the amount of carbohydrate eaten, the greater the rise in blood glucose levels. Advice on the correct amount of carbohydrate at mealtimes varies amongst health professionals, but what has been used in practice with success is aiming for around 40g carbs at meals and 10-15g carbs for snacks.

Your dietitian or healthcare professional will discuss portion sizes with you. Most recipes in this book have been developed to contain around 40g carbs or less. Where there are recipes containing more than 40g carbs, rest assured that the carbohydrates in these meals are slow releasing and therefore will have minimal impact on your blood glucose levels.

Please note: Fruit is encouraged in the diet but it is important to be aware of the high natural sugar content. Despite being low in calories and fat, most fruits are high in carbohydrate and therefore portion control is important. 3 or 4 portions of fruit, spread over the day, is a good guide.

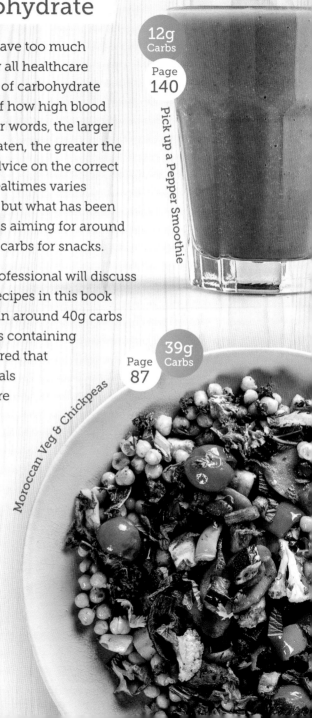

12g Carbs

Page 140

Pick up a Pepper Smoothie

39g Carbs

Page 87

Moroccan Veg & Chickpeas

West African & Afro-Caribbean Foods

Some food cultures such as African and Caribbean cuisine are very diverse, but one thing common in all is the heavy dependence on starchy carbs. The amount of carbohydrates eaten at a meal or as a snack, as mentioned on the previous page, is very important, as is the Glycaemic Index.

The images below show food and drinks commonly consumed that are known to have a big impact on blood glucose levels, and therefore should be avoided or their consumption significantly reduced.

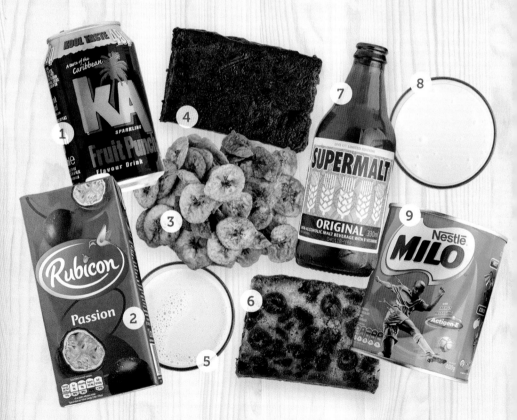

1. KA
2. Rubicon
3. Plantain chips
4. Caribbean sweet bread
5. Evaporated milk
6. Jamaican fruit bread
7. Supermalt
8. Condensed milk
9. Milo

Tips for controlling your blood glucose levels

High-five to healthy fats!

Fat does not cause your blood glucose levels to rise and will help to keep you feeling full. Avocados, nuts and seeds, oily fish such as salmon or mackerel, olive and rapeseed oil are all examples of unsaturated fats (the 'healthy fats').

Prioritise high quality, lean protein sources

These include lean meat, poultry, fish, eggs, cheese, pulses, nuts and seeds, which are known to have minimal impact on your blood glucose levels but keep you feeling full for longer. You will be advised to reduce your carbohydrate intake, so make sure you have a protein portion at every meal. You could, for example, add nuts and seeds to your breakfast bowl.

Reach for the rainbow!

Fruit and veg should be a staple in your diet and variety is important. Fruit has natural sugars that can cause blood glucose levels to rise, so limit yourself to a portion at a time (e.g. an apple or orange as a snack instead of a large bowl of fruit salad). Vegetables can be eaten to your heart's content, as they have little impact on your blood glucose levels and contain fibre to aid a healthy bowel and keep you feeling full. See Meal Plan 5 on page 44 to see how easy it is to reach 10½ fruit & veg portions per day and still keep your carb intake in check!

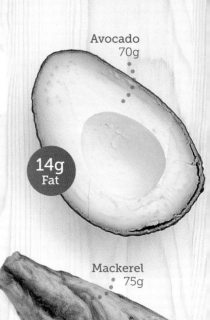

Avocado
70g

14g
Fat

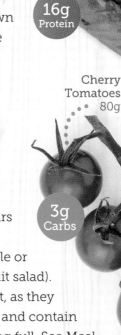

Mackerel
75g

16g
Protein

Cherry
Tomatoes
80g

3g
Carbs

Start the day the right way!

Most breakfast products on the market are high in carbs and low in protein, so are therefore unlikely to keep you satisfied until your next meal. Stay fuller for longer with these simple swaps:

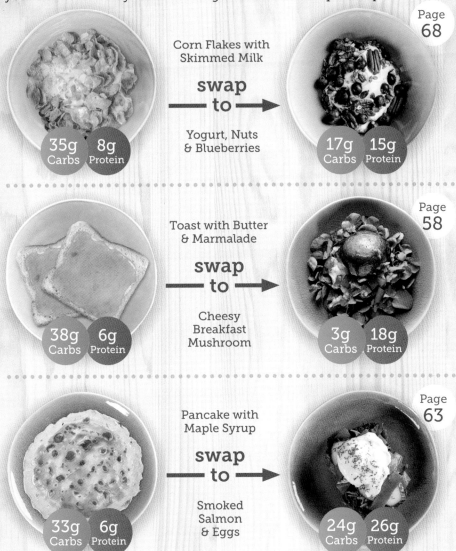

Page **68**

Corn Flakes with
Skimmed Milk

swap to →

Yogurt, Nuts
& Blueberries

35g Carbs 8g Protein

17g Carbs 15g Protein

Page **58**

Toast with Butter
& Marmalade

swap to →

Cheesy
Breakfast
Mushroom

38g Carbs 6g Protein

3g Carbs 18g Protein

Page **63**

Pancake with
Maple Syrup

swap to →

Smoked
Salmon
& Eggs

33g Carbs 6g Protein

24g Carbs 26g Protein

Please note: Some of the swaps are low in carbohydrate and you may need to add additional carbs if you are taking insulin, to avoid hypoglycaemia. If unsure, discuss this with your healthcare team.

Include lentils and pulses in your meals

Fibre recommendations have been increased to 30g per day and a great way to achieve this is by boosting your bean intake. Beans and pulses (such as chickpeas, lentils and butter beans) count towards your 5-a-day, are high in fibre and known to release energy slowly; great if you are getting the munchies between meals. Try adding chickpeas to your salad, replacing rice with puy lentils or simply adding lentils to your beef stew. Thanks to brilliant beans and pulses, a couple of our daily meal plans boast a whopping 40g fibre per day!

Kidney Beans 80g

7g Fibre

Limit your intake of sugars

Avoid added or naturally-occurring sugars from products like fruit juice (homemade and shop bought), sweetened drinks (such as squash, fizzy drinks or sports drinks), desserts, honey, maple syrup and dried fruit.

3 Cals

Squash (no added sugar) Half Pint

Get savvy with your snacks

Rather than 2 or 3 main meals with large portions of carbohydrate, try to spread your carb intake throughout the day. If you are reducing your carbs at meals, you are likely to get hungry before your next meal. Snacks that include protein and carbohydrate will halt those hunger pangs with little effect on your blood glucose levels. For some great snack suggestions, see pages 134 to 143.

Cheesy Oatcakes

Page 141

15g Carbs

7g Protein

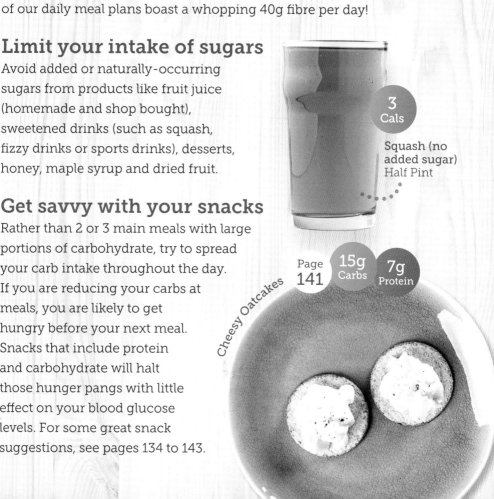

Get creative with your carbs!

Try replacing your usual carbohydrate choices with lower carb alternatives, such as:

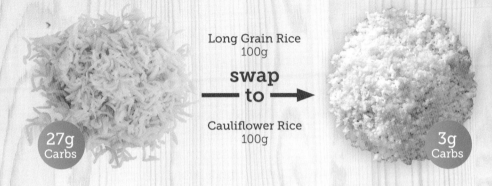

Long Grain Rice
100g

**swap
to** →

Cauliflower Rice
100g

27g
Carbs

3g
Carbs

Other healthy eating considerations during pregnancy

Weight changes

For some women, a diagnosis of gestational diabetes can mean a few small changes to their diet and physical activity levels, whilst for others it requires a complete diet and lifestyle overhaul. Portion sizes, drinks, snack choices and physical activity need re-evaluating, which can lead to weight loss or smaller weight gains than expected. But what is an expected amount of weight gain during pregnancy? Healthcare professionals, family members and peers all influence our expectations on what a 'healthy weight gain' should be, but is there such a thing?

Currently in the UK there are no formal evidence-based guidelines on what a 'healthy weight gain' during pregnancy should be. Factors contributing to weight gain include the weight of the unborn child, placenta, amniotic fluid, increases in maternal blood and fluid volume, as well as increased maternal body fat (stored for breastfeeding). Whilst most women put on some weight in pregnancy, every woman is different and the above factors mean that weight gain can vary a great deal.

The National Institute for Health and Clinical Excellence (NICE) developed some guidelines in 2010 which stated:

★ Dieting during pregnancy is not recommended as it may harm the health of the unborn child.

★ There is no need to 'eat for two' or to drink whole milk.

Whilst pregnancy is not a time for trying to lose weight, it is a time to place greater focus on eating the right foods and staying active. For women who make healthy changes to their diet and lifestyle to manage their gestational diabetes (e.g. increasing physical activity levels or choosing healthier snack choices), this can result in smaller weight gains. Equally, putting on too much weight due to calorie excess can lead to health problems for you and your unborn baby. Historically, women were encouraged to 'eat for two' resulting in higher calorie intakes and greater weight gains. We now know this is unnecessary and calorie requirements increase only slightly in the last 3 months (and then only by around 200 calories per day).

If you have concerns, speak with the healthcare team that is monitoring you and your baby regularly during your pregnancy.

Vitamin supplements

Eating a healthy, varied diet will ensure you get most of the vitamins and minerals you need. However, during pregnancy your requirements for some nutrients increase (including vitamin D and folic acid), whilst too much vitamin A could be harmful to your baby.

You can get specific multivitamins for pregnancy from pharmacies and supermarkets, or your GP may be able to prescribe them for you. If you wish to continue with a standard multivitamin tablet, make sure that the tablet does not contain vitamin A (or retinol). Fish liver oil supplements should not be taken whilst pregnant.

Some women may be eligible for free vitamins through the Government's Healthy Start scheme. Talk to your GP or midwife for further information.

Iron

Some women find that their iron levels are low during pregnancy, which can cause tiredness and anaemia. Pregnancy blood tests can show if your iron levels are low. Iron rich foods include red meat, leafy green vegetables, eggs, and nuts. Additionally, many breakfast cereals are fortified, meaning that they have added vitamins and minerals to boost their nutritional content. Vitamin C (from fruit and vegetables) helps the absorption of iron whilst a cup of tea can reduce it.

If you are diagnosed with anaemia, your midwife or GP will advise that you start taking an iron supplement. Many women are often encouraged to take their tablet in the morning with a glass of fruit juice (which we know will cause your blood glucose levels to rise). Therefore, a good alternative is to take it with a glass of water.

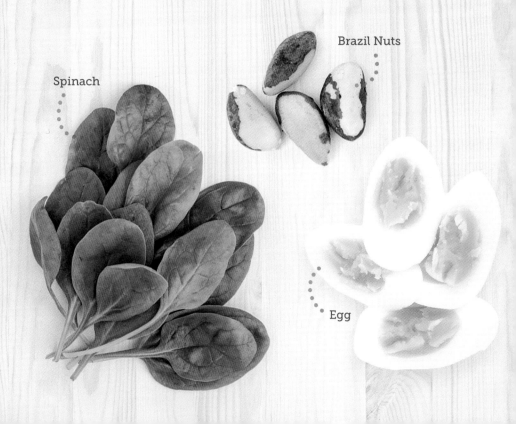

Brazil Nuts

Spinach

Egg

Calcium

Together with vitamin D, calcium is important for the development and maintenance of healthy, strong bones and teeth. It is a nutrient needed by both mother and baby. Whilst calcium requirements do not increase during pregnancy, it is important to ensure your diet contains sufficient calcium.

Dairy foods such as milk, cheese and yogurt are rich sources of calcium. Other good sources include calcium enriched non-dairy milk alternatives such as almond, soya, coconut and rice milk, fish with small edible bones such as mackerel, dried apricots, almonds and green leafy vegetables including broccoli.

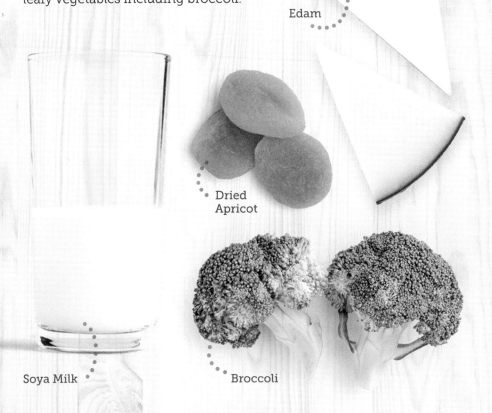

Edam

Dried Apricot

Soya Milk

Broccoli

Nuts

The latest guidance for mothers who would like to eat peanuts (or foods containing peanuts) during pregnancy or breastfeeding is they can choose to do so as part of a healthy balanced diet, irrespective of whether they have a family history of allergies. Anyone with an allergy should continue to avoid peanuts.

Food safety

Some foods, such as pâté, undercooked meat/fish and some cheeses, are advised to be avoided whilst pregnant, as they might make you ill or harm your baby. For more information, please discuss with your healthcare professional or visit NHS Choices: www.nhs.uk

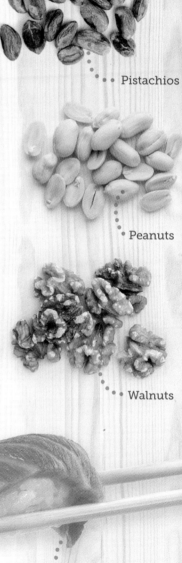

Pistachios

Peanuts

Walnuts

Pâté

Salmon Nigiri

Stilton

What can I drink?

It is all too easy to forget the importance of drinking when you are focusing on what you can and can't eat. Drinking enough fluids can help with some common pregnancy problems, such as constipation, swelling and tiredness. A good guide is to aim for 8 medium glasses (200ml per glass) each day.

Good choices include:

★ Water (still or sparkling)

★ Coffee / tea (normal and decaf - see caffeine guidance opposite)

★ Fresh milk

★ Non-dairy milk alternatives, such as almond, soya, coconut, rice

★ Fruit teas

★ No added sugar squash / fizzy drinks

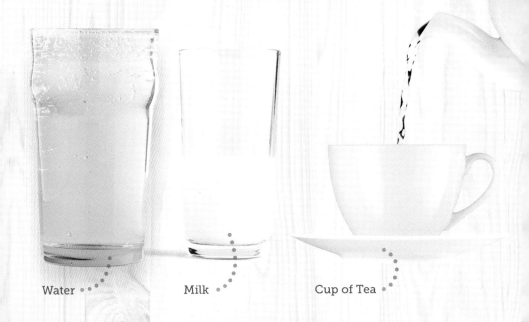

Water   Milk   Cup of Tea

Caffeine

It is important to limit the amount of caffeine in your diet, as too much caffeine has been shown to increase the risk of babies born with a low birth weight (which can cause health problems later in life). High levels of caffeine might also cause a miscarriage. You don't need to cut out caffeine completely, and don't worry if you occasionally have too much as the risks are likely to be very small. The current guidance is to limit your intake to 200mg caffeine per day.

The amount of caffeine in food and drinks will vary but the following is a guide:

★ 2 mugs of instant coffee (100mg each)

★ 1 mug of filter coffee (140mg each)

★ 2 mugs of tea (75mg each)

★ 5 cans of cola* (up to 40mg each)

★ 2 cans of energy drink* (up to 80mg each)

★ 4 (50g) bars of plain chocolate* (up to 50 mg each)

* **Please note:** these products are also high in sugar.

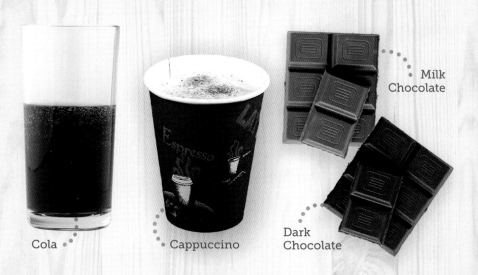

Cola

Cappuccino

Milk Chocolate

Dark Chocolate

How to use this book

This book includes 80 carefully-created recipes (plus 20 snacks) for mealtimes across the day, divided into the following sections:

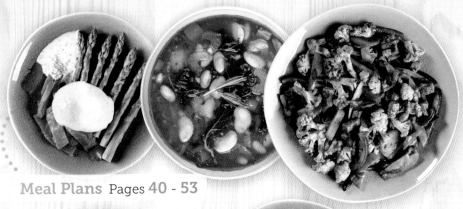

Meal Plans Pages **40 - 53**

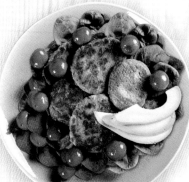

Recipes
Pages **54 - 133**

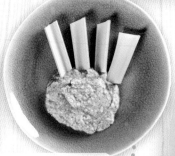

Snacks
Pages **134 - 143**

Individual Foods Pages **144 - 215**

Within each section, the recipes are listed in calorie order, starting with the lowest calorie recipe. For each dish, the nutritional information for the following nutrients are clearly displayed in colour coded circles:

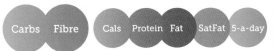

Carbs Fibre   Cals Protein Fat SatFat 5-a-day

Simply browse the variety of recipes and select ones that meet your dietary goal.

Recipes

The first part of the book contains 80 recipes to prepare and enjoy, with knowledge that your meal choices are in line with the nutritional guidelines for gestational diabetes. Most meals contain less than 40g carbs and all use good quality protein and low GI carbohydrate sources, to help minimise any rises in blood glucose levels. Those that have more than 40g carbs have a low GI, so a greater allowance of carbohydrate has been given in some cases. Each recipe is for 1 portion, but can be doubled up or made into larger quantities and portioned out.

At the back of the book, there is a visual guide showing the portion sizes of commonly consumed foods. This offers you the flexibility to pick and choose what carbohydrate to eat with your meals. Please note, however, that some meals will already contain 40g carbs per portion, so there is no further 'allowance' for additional carbohydrate.

Breakfast is a time when we can be more resistant to insulin due to hormones, and even small amounts of carbs cause a significant rise in blood glucose levels. Therefore, many of our breakfast options are low in carbohydrate. Should you be able to tolerate carbs, extra can be eaten (for example, in Meal Plan 7 baked beans could be added to the omelette, or bread could be added to Avocado & Eggs in Meal Plan 3).

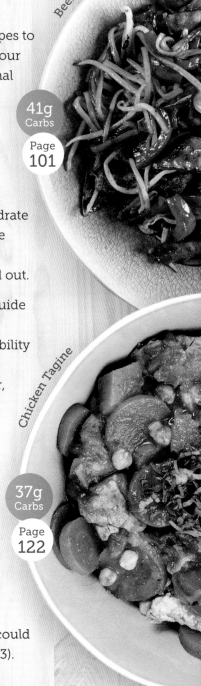

Beef Lo Mein

41g
Carbs

Page
101

Chicken Tagine

37g
Carbs

Page
122

Meal Plans

We've devised some daily meal plans to offer you some ideas on how to reduce your carbohydrate intake but still eat tasty, nutritious meals according to your dietary preferences. All plans include a breakfast, lunch and evening meal idea, with some offering extra carb food suggestions for meals.

41g Carbs

Page **70**

Fruity Porridge

30g Carbs

Page **114**

48g Carbs

Page **78**

Okra & Lentil Curry

Warm Squash Salad

Snacks

Mozzarella & Tomato

This book also contains a separate snack section. To ensure you consume adequate energy and nutrients, you are encouraged to choose 2-3 snacks per day. Some meal plans include snack suggestions, which can be swapped according to personal preference. All snacks are under 15g carbs and many include protein to help control blood glucose and hunger levels.

6g Carbs

Page **142**

Individual foods

If you already know your way around the kitchen and have recipes you want to use, then turn to the back of the book for a list of ingredients. The nutritional content of each individual ingredient is shown, giving you the flexibility to build your own recipes. This visual method allows you to quickly select foods in appropriate portions to develop your own meal plans. You may find it useful to write down the details of your creations so you have a record of the nutritional information and can make the recipe again in future.

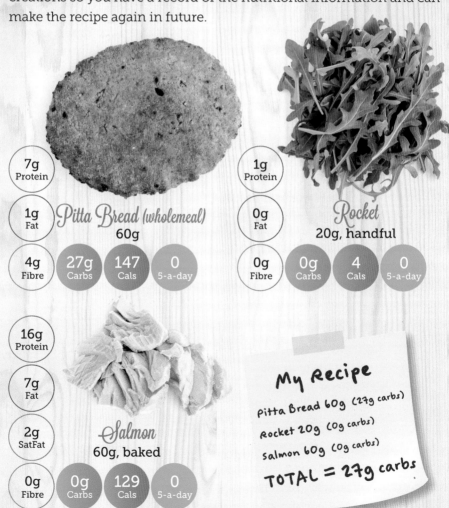

Pitta Bread (wholemeal)
60g

7g Protein
1g Fat
4g Fibre
27g Carbs
147 Cals
0 5-a-day

Rocket
20g, handful

1g Protein
0g Fat
0g Fibre
0g Carbs
4 Cals
0 5-a-day

Salmon
60g, baked

16g Protein
7g Fat
2g SatFat
0g Fibre
0g Carbs
129 Cals
0 5-a-day

My Recipe

Pitta Bread 60g (27g carbs)

Rocket 20g (0g carbs)

Salmon 60g (0g carbs)

TOTAL = 27g carbs

A few things to note:

★ Planning ahead is key to success. Try to make time each week to write a shopping list and plan for all the meals and snacks you will eat that week.

★ Consider cooking in bulk. This is a great way to always have a meal in the fridge or freezer and to save money. Most of the recipes in this book can be cooked in bulk.

★ The recipes use average/medium sizes of vegetables and fruit, and weights shown are for the edible part (after being peeled or stoned), unless otherwise stated.

★ Some recipes use a handy measure (e.g. 'large handful of watercress') instead of a specific weight. Should you wish to know the exact weight, simply find that portion in the ingredients section. For example, the Quinoa Stuffed Mushrooms recipe on page 83 uses '1 large handful Watercress'. Looking at watercress on page 213, you will see that 1 large handful weighs 20g.

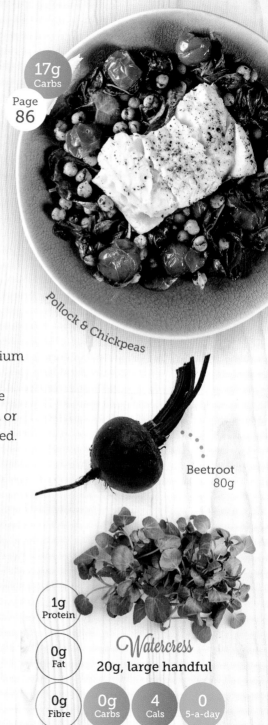

17g Carbs

Page 86

Pollock & Chickpeas

Beetroot 80g

1g Protein

0g Fat

0g Fibre

Watercress
20g, large handful

0g Carbs

4 Cals

0 5-a-day

★ Other cuts of meat and/or fish can be used in the recipes without changing the carb content (although the calorie and fat content will probably change).

★ If you like your dish spicier, or love the flavour of fresh mint, you can be heavy handed and add more to your taste. Adding these herbs and spices will not affect the carb content.

1
Cal

Rosemary Sprig

★ Not all the recipes include salt and pepper, so adding such seasoning is down to personal preference. Such addition will not affect the carb content.

★ The recipes use a mix of uncooked and cooked weights for rice, pasta, couscous, quinoa and pearl barley. The table below outlines the simple conversion for uncooked and cooked weights, although please bear in mind that the longer you cook your pasta and rice, the more water it absorbs, which will affect the final weight of the cooked product.

	Uncooked Weight	Cooked Weight
Couscous	35g	80g
Dried Pasta	45g	100g
Pearl Barley	25g	80g
Quinoa	30g	80g
Rice	35g	100g

White Fusilli Pasta 100g

Pearl Barley 80g

Buying ingredients

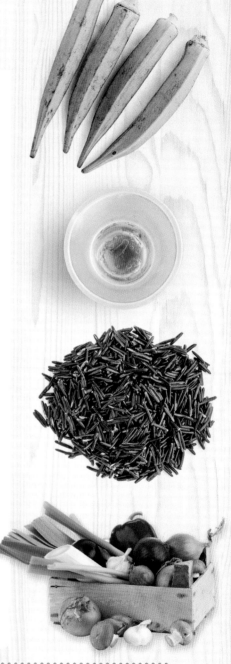

★ It is best to use wholegrain pasta and rice to boost fibre content.

★ Use olive oil where possible. Alternatives include rapeseed and groundnut (peanut) oil.

★ Where possible, use fresh, ripe fruit & vegetables.

★ Use good quality, organic produce as often as possible.

★ To keep the cost down, choose vegetables and fruit that are in season. Alternatively, you can replace one vegetable with another that is in season, but be mindful this may change the nutritional content.

★ The thickness of shop bought tahini paste can vary, so you may wish to add more water to achieve the desired consistency.

★ A great way to add variety to your diet and ensure you always have your ingredients to hand is to order a fruit and vegetable box. Each delivery is different so you will receive a variety of different ingredients!

To see our recommended veg box companies, please visit:
www.carbsandcals.com/vegbox

Cooking Glossary

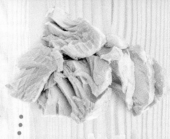

Blanch: Briefly cook vegetables in boiling water to seal in flavour and colour.

Drizzle: Pour a small amount of liquid (e.g. dressing) onto food item or salad.

Flake: Use a fork, or hand, to break cooked fish into smaller pieces and to check if the fish is cooked. If cooked, the flesh should fall away easily.

Matchstick: Cut into thin strips.

Mince: Chop very finely.

Parboil: Boil ingredient until it is partially cooked.

Ribbon: Shave vegetables into ribbons using a peeler. If you have a spiralizer, this would work just as well.

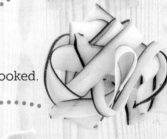

Sauté: From the French verb, sauter, meaning 'to jump'. Sautéed food is cooked in a small amount of fat in an open pan on a high heat.

Segment: Divide citrus fruit into smaller sections.

Thinly slice: Slice ingredient into thin slices using a sharp knife or spiralizer.

Toasted nuts: Nuts heated in a medium-hot frying pan (without the addition of oil) to bring out the richness and flavour. Toast for a couple of minutes until fragrant, or light brown in colour.

What next?

5g
Carbs

Satsuma
80g

Breastfeeding

The benefits of breastfeeding are well known and women with diabetes are still able, and are encouraged, to breastfeed. After delivery, most women with gestational diabetes will be advised to stop their diabetes medication and their blood glucose levels will be monitored. The change in hormone levels after birth means insulin requirements drop significantly.

For women with type 1 and type 2 diabetes, breastfeeding can lower your insulin requirements further (by up to 25%). Breast milk contains the sugar lactose, therefore each time you breastfeed you lose some lactose, which means your blood glucose levels drop. This can be managed by changing your medication doses (on advice from your healthcare team) or having a small snack containing carbohydrate when you breastfeed, for example a milky drink, piece of fruit or a small cereal bar.

Speak with your healthcare team for further information on medication changes and doses when breastfeeding.

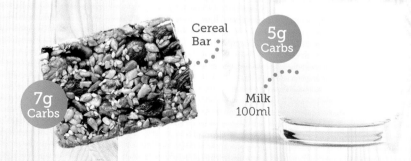

Cereal
Bar

5g
Carbs

7g
Carbs

Milk
100ml

Long term implications

After pregnancy, most women diagnosed with gestational diabetes find that the diabetes disappears. However, a small percentage continue to experience high blood glucose levels and may be diagnosed with type 2 diabetes.

Research has shown that women with gestational diabetes have an increased risk of developing type 2 diabetes. In fact, 50-60% go on to develop type 2, with a peak in the five years following childbirth.

Fortunately, you can act now to prevent or delay the onset of diabetes by following a few simple rules:

★ Eat well and achieve a healthy weight.
★ Be active.
★ Have your blood glucose level measured every year.
★ Be aware of the symptoms of diabetes, such as excessive thirst, needing to go to the toilet a lot, tiredness and/or unexplained weight loss.
★ If you become pregnant in the future, always inform your GP and midwife about your previous diagnosis of gestational diabetes.

For more support and guidance on healthy eating and weight loss, check out our other books & app:

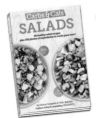 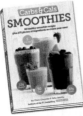 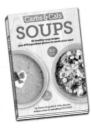 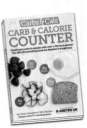 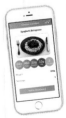

www.carbsandcals.com

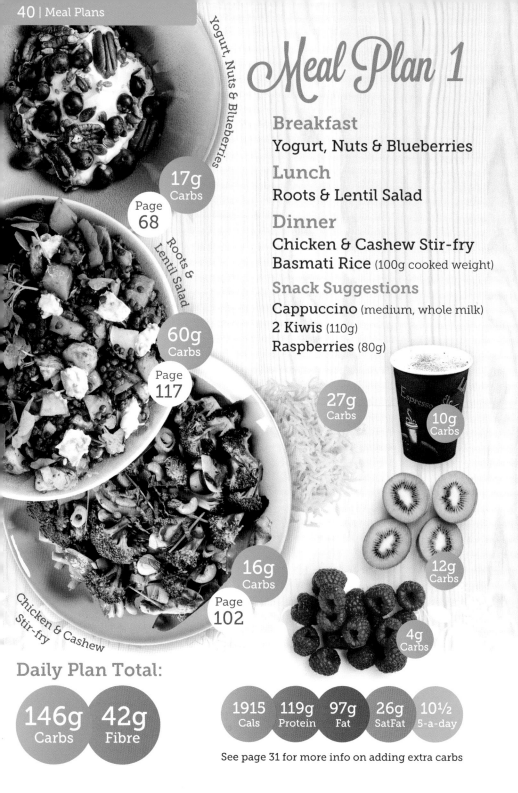

Yogurt, Nuts & Blueberries

Meal Plan 1

Breakfast
Yogurt, Nuts & Blueberries

Lunch
Roots & Lentil Salad

Dinner
Chicken & Cashew Stir-fry
Basmati Rice (100g cooked weight)

Snack Suggestions
Cappuccino (medium, whole milk)
2 Kiwis (110g)
Raspberries (80g)

17g Carbs

Page **68**

Roots & Lentil Salad

60g Carbs

Page **117**

27g Carbs

10g Carbs

Chicken & Cashew Stir-fry

16g Carbs

Page **102**

12g Carbs

4g Carbs

Daily Plan Total:

146g Carbs

42g Fibre

| 1915 Cals | 119g Protein | 97g Fat | 26g SatFat | 10½ 5-a-day |

See page 31 for more info on adding extra carbs

Meal Plan 2

Breakfast
Cheesy Breakfast Mushroom
Avofennel Smoothie

Lunch
Tuna & Bean Salad
Granary Bread (with 1 tsp butter)

Dinner
Dijon Chicken with Mash
Vanilla Berries
Greek Yogurt (100g)

Snack Suggestions
Milk (half pint, semi-skimmed)
Orange (140g, small)
Almonds (3 tbsp)

3g Carbs
Page **58**
Cheesy Breakfast Mushroom

20g Carbs

17g Carbs
Page **111**
Tuna & Bean Salad

11g Carbs
Page **140**
Avofennel Smoothie

29g Carbs
Page **106**

13g Carbs

8g Carbs

2g Carbs

5g Carbs

13g Carbs
Page **135**
Vanilla Berries

Dijon Chicken with Mash

Daily Plan Total:

12½ 5-a-day
38g SatFat
103g Fat
157g Protein
2035 Cals

39g Fibre
121g Carbs

See page 31 for more info on adding extra carbs

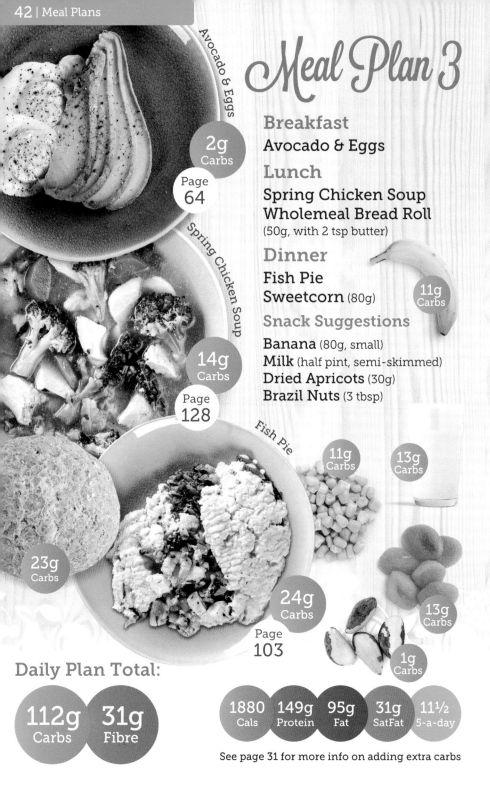

Avocado & Eggs

Meal Plan 3

Breakfast
Avocado & Eggs

2g Carbs

Page 64

Lunch
Spring Chicken Soup
Wholemeal Bread Roll
(50g, with 2 tsp butter)

Dinner
Fish Pie
Sweetcorn (80g)

11g Carbs

Snack Suggestions
Banana (80g, small)
Milk (half pint, semi-skimmed)
Dried Apricots (30g)
Brazil Nuts (3 tbsp)

Spring Chicken Soup

14g Carbs

Page 128

Fish Pie

11g Carbs

13g Carbs

23g Carbs

24g Carbs

Page 103

13g Carbs

1g Carbs

Daily Plan Total:

112g Carbs   31g Fibre

1880 Cals   149g Protein   95g Fat   31g SatFat   11½ 5-a-day

See page 31 for more info on adding extra carbs

Meal Plan 4

Breakfast
Fruity Porridge

Lunch
Kale Kerfuffle Smoothie
Warm Squash Salad

Dinner
Okra & Lentil Curry

Snack Suggestions
Blackberries (160g)
Greek Yogurt (200g)
Cheesy Oatcakes

41g Carbs

Page **70**

Fruity Porridge

48g Carbs

Page **78**

Okra & Lentil Curry

10g Carbs

Kale Kerfuffle Smoothie

30g Carbs

Page **114**

Warm Squash Salad

8g Carbs

15g Carbs

Page **141**

17g Carbs

Page **54**

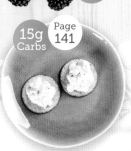

12½ 5-a-day **31g** SatFat **102g** Fat **73g** Protein **1850** Cals

Daily Plan Total:

49g Fibre **169g** Carbs

See page 31 for more info on adding extra carbs

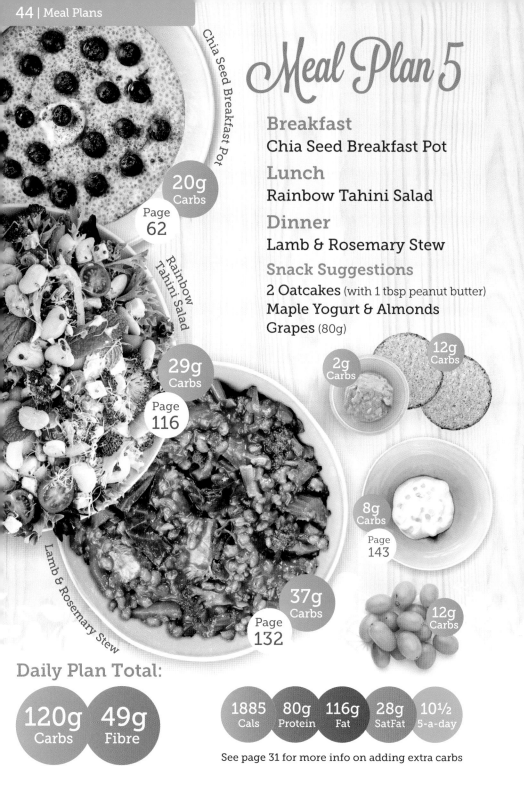

Chia Seed Breakfast Pot

Meal Plan 5

20g Carbs

Page **62**

Rainbow Tahini Salad

Breakfast
Chia Seed Breakfast Pot

Lunch
Rainbow Tahini Salad

Dinner
Lamb & Rosemary Stew

Snack Suggestions
2 Oatcakes (with 1 tbsp peanut butter)
Maple Yogurt & Almonds
Grapes (80g)

29g Carbs

Page **116**

2g Carbs

12g Carbs

8g Carbs

Page **143**

Lamb & Rosemary Stew

37g Carbs

Page **132**

12g Carbs

Daily Plan Total:

120g Carbs

49g Fibre

| 1885 Cals | 80g Protein | 116g Fat | 28g SatFat | 10½ 5-a-day |

See page 31 for more info on adding extra carbs

Meal Plan 6

Breakfast
Cauli Smoothie

Lunch
Salmon Kebabs
Quinoa (160g cooked weight)

Dinner
Mexican Chicken Mole
Guacamole

Snack Suggestions
Raspberries (80g)
Greek Yogurt (100g)
Walnuts (3 tbsp)

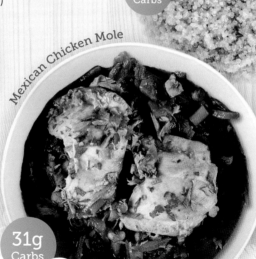

Salmon Kebabs

Cauli Smoothie

21g Carbs

Page 55

30g Carbs

Page 100

13g Carbs

Mexican Chicken Mole

4g Carbs

5g Carbs

1g Carbs

31g Carbs

Page 104

6g Carbs

Page 142

Daily Plan Total:

15 5-a-day	22g SatFat	102g Fat	113g Protein	1825 Cals

39g Fibre

111g Carbs

See page 31 for more info on adding extra carbs

Mushroom Pepper Omelette

6g Carbs
Page 67

Carrot & Lentil Soup

34g Carbs
Page 125

27g Carbs

6g Carbs
Page 107

Chicken, Kale & Chorizo

30g Carbs

Meal Plan 7

Breakfast
Mushroom Pepper Omelette

Lunch
Carrot & Lentil Soup
Wholemeal Pitta Bread (60g)

Dinner
Chicken, Kale & Chorizo
New Potatoes (200g)

Snack Suggestions
Mozzarella & Tomato
Spicy Chickpeas
2 Figs (60g)

6g Carbs
Page 142

14g Carbs
Page 143

6g Carbs

Daily Plan Total:

129g Carbs

32g Fibre

1975 Cals

116g Protein

110g Fat

37g SatFat

9 5-a-day

See page 31 for more info on adding extra carbs

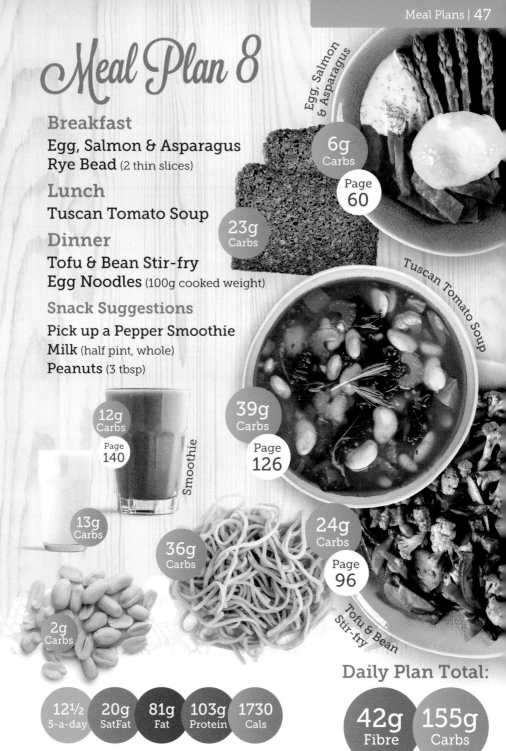

Meal Plan 8

Breakfast
Egg, Salmon & Asparagus
Rye Bead (2 thin slices)

Lunch
Tuscan Tomato Soup

Dinner
Tofu & Bean Stir-fry
Egg Noodles (100g cooked weight)

Snack Suggestions
Pick up a Pepper Smoothie
Milk (half pint, whole)
Peanuts (3 tbsp)

Egg, Salmon & Asparagus

6g Carbs

Page **60**

23g Carbs

Tuscan Tomato Soup

Smoothie

12g Carbs

Page **140**

39g Carbs

Page **126**

13g Carbs

36g Carbs

24g Carbs

Page **96**

Tofu & Bean Stir-fry

2g Carbs

12½ 5-a-day

20g SatFat

81g Fat

103g Protein

1730 Cals

Daily Plan Total:

42g Fibre

155g Carbs

See page 31 for more info on adding extra carbs

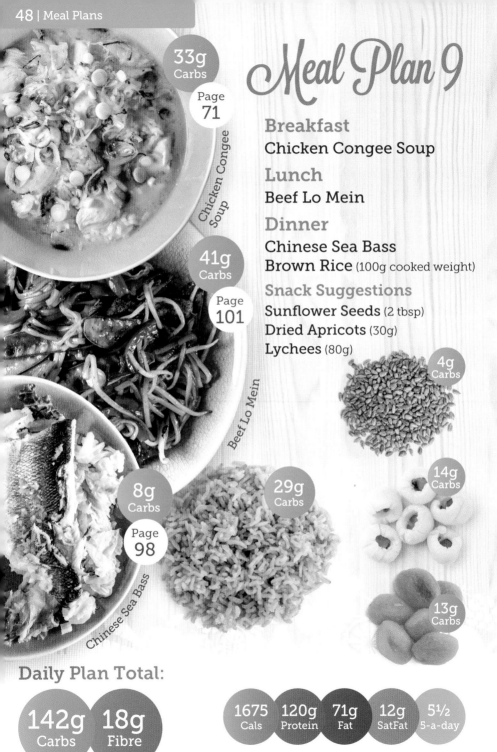

Meal Plan 9

Breakfast
Chicken Congee Soup

Lunch
Beef Lo Mein

Dinner
Chinese Sea Bass
Brown Rice (100g cooked weight)

Snack Suggestions
Sunflower Seeds (2 tbsp)
Dried Apricots (30g)
Lychees (80g)

33g Carbs

Page 71

Chicken Congee Soup

41g Carbs

Page 101

Beef Lo Mein

8g Carbs

Page 98

Chinese Sea Bass

29g Carbs

4g Carbs

14g Carbs

13g Carbs

Daily Plan Total:

142g Carbs

18g Fibre

1675 Cals

120g Protein

71g Fat

12g SatFat

5½ 5-a-day

See page 31 for more info on adding extra carbs

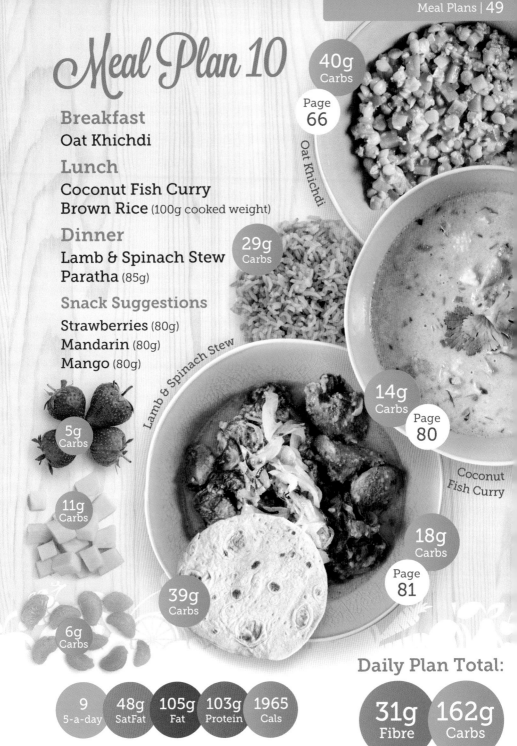

Meal Plan 10

Breakfast
Oat Khichdi

Lunch
Coconut Fish Curry
Brown Rice (100g cooked weight)

Dinner
Lamb & Spinach Stew
Paratha (85g)

Snack Suggestions
Strawberries (80g)
Mandarin (80g)
Mango (80g)

40g Carbs

Page 66

Oat Khichdi

29g Carbs

14g Carbs

Page 80

5g Carbs

11g Carbs

18g Carbs

Page 81

39g Carbs

6g Carbs

Lamb & Spinach Stew

Coconut Fish Curry

Daily Plan Total:

9 5-a-day
48g SatFat
105g Fat
103g Protein
1965 Cals

31g Fibre
162g Carbs

See page 31 for more info on adding extra carbs

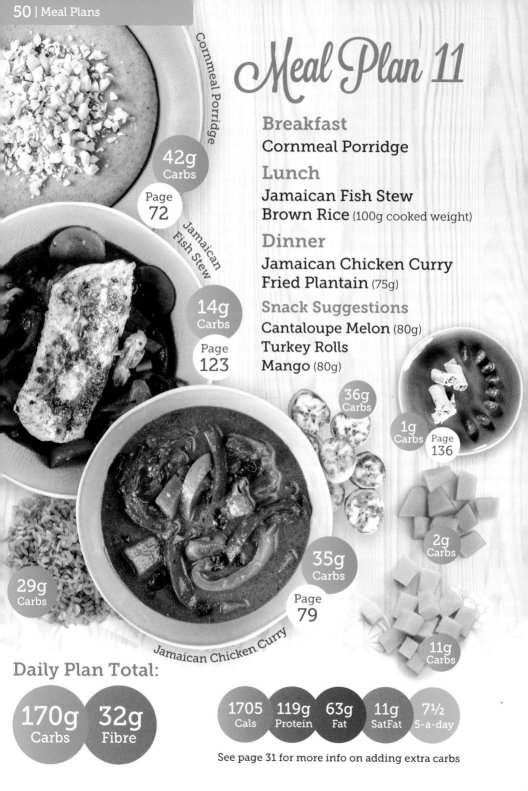

Cornmeal Porridge

Meal Plan 11

Breakfast
Cornmeal Porridge

Lunch
Jamaican Fish Stew
Brown Rice (100g cooked weight)

Dinner
Jamaican Chicken Curry
Fried Plantain (75g)

Snack Suggestions
Cantaloupe Melon (80g)
Turkey Rolls
Mango (80g)

42g Carbs
Page **72**

Jamaican Fish Stew

14g Carbs
Page **123**

36g Carbs

1g Carbs
Page **136**

2g Carbs

35g Carbs
Page **79**

29g Carbs

11g Carbs

Jamaican Chicken Curry

Daily Plan Total:

170g Carbs **32g** Fibre

1705 Cals **119g** Protein **63g** Fat **11g** SatFat **7½** 5-a-day

See page 31 for more info on adding extra carbs

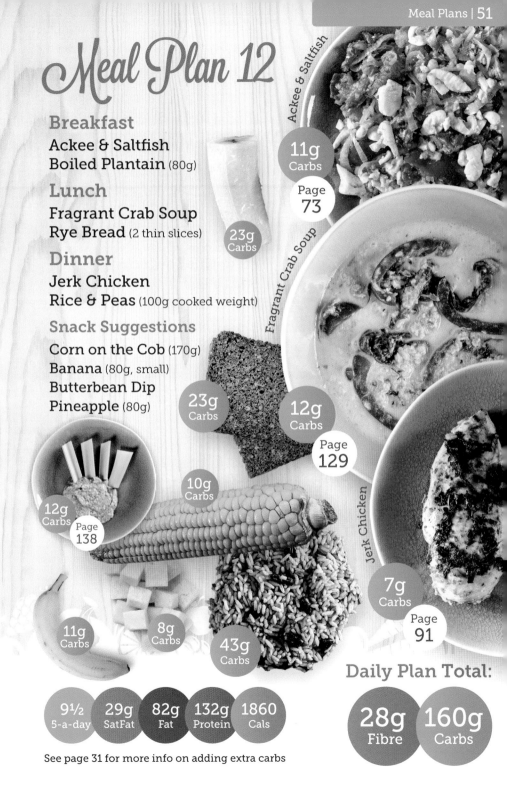

Meal Plan 12

Breakfast

Ackee & Saltfish
Boiled Plantain (80g)

Lunch

Fragrant Crab Soup
Rye Bread (2 thin slices)

Dinner

Jerk Chicken
Rice & Peas (100g cooked weight)

Snack Suggestions

Corn on the Cob (170g)
Banana (80g, small)
Butterbean Dip
Pineapple (80g)

Ackee & Saltfish

11g Carbs
Page **73**

Fragrant Crab Soup

23g Carbs

23g Carbs

12g Carbs
Page **129**

10g Carbs

12g Carbs
Page **138**

Jerk Chicken

7g Carbs
Page **91**

11g Carbs

8g Carbs

43g Carbs

Daily Plan Total:

9½ 5-a-day
29g SatFat
82g Fat
132g Protein
1860 Cals

28g Fibre
160g Carbs

See page 31 for more info on adding extra carbs

Eggs & Fried Plantain

Meal Plan 13

Breakfast
Eggs & Fried Plantain

38g Carbs

Page **69**

Lunch
Nigerian Chicken Stew
Boiled Yam (100g)

Dinner
Palm Nut Soup
Fufu (100g)

Snack Suggestions
Dried Apricots (30g)
Papaya (120g)
Plum (90g)

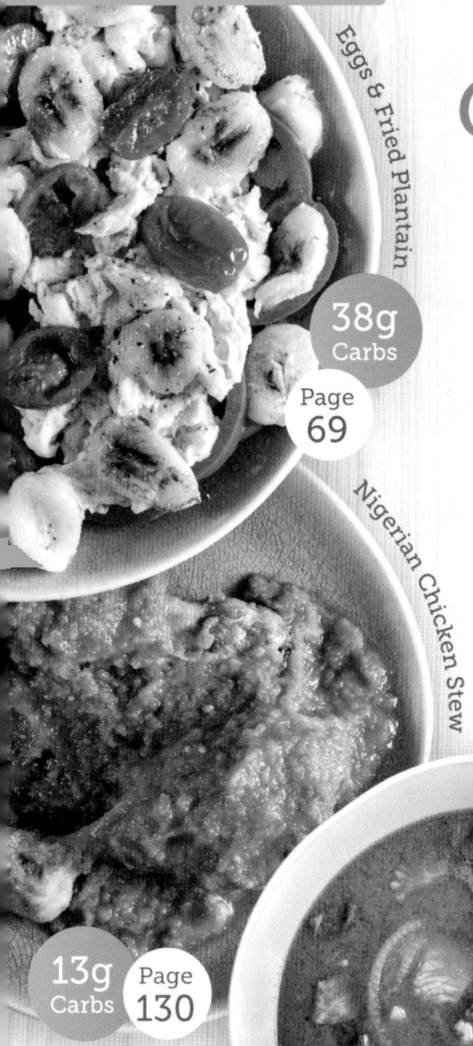

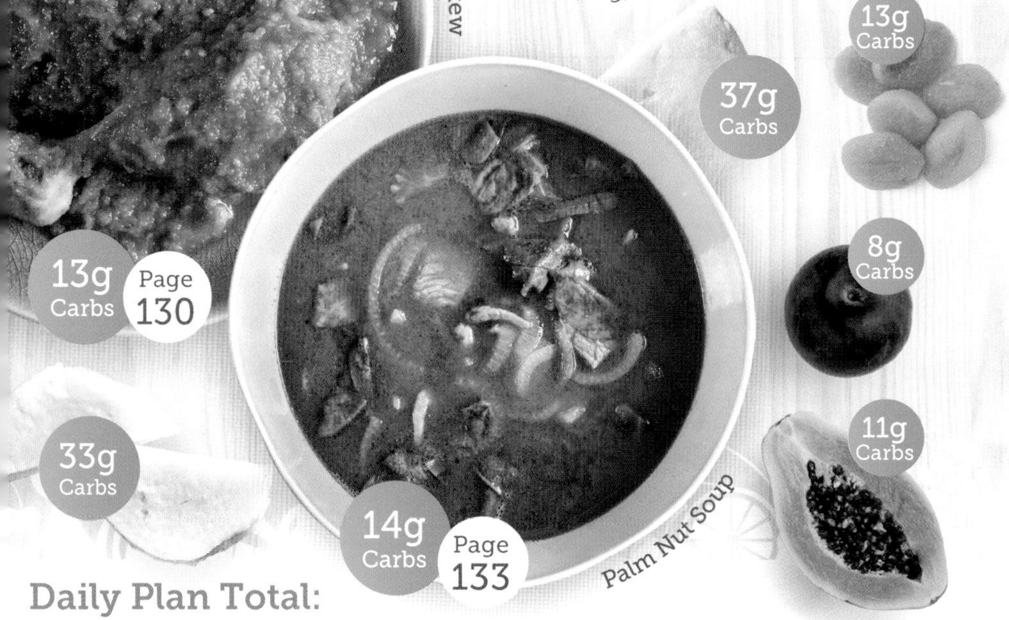

Nigerian Chicken Stew

13g Carbs

37g Carbs

13g Carbs Page **130**

8g Carbs

33g Carbs

14g Carbs Page **133**

11g Carbs

Palm Nut Soup

Daily Plan Total:

167g Carbs

24g Fibre

1930 Cals

96g Protein

101g Fat

17g SatFat

9 5-a-day

See page 31 for more info on adding extra carbs

Meal Plan 14

Breakfast
Sardines with Salad

Lunch
Groundnut Soup
Fufu (100g)

Dinner
African Bean Stew
Fried Plantain (75g)

Snack Suggestions
Tuna Lettuce Wraps
Milk (half pint, whole)
Watermelon (80g)

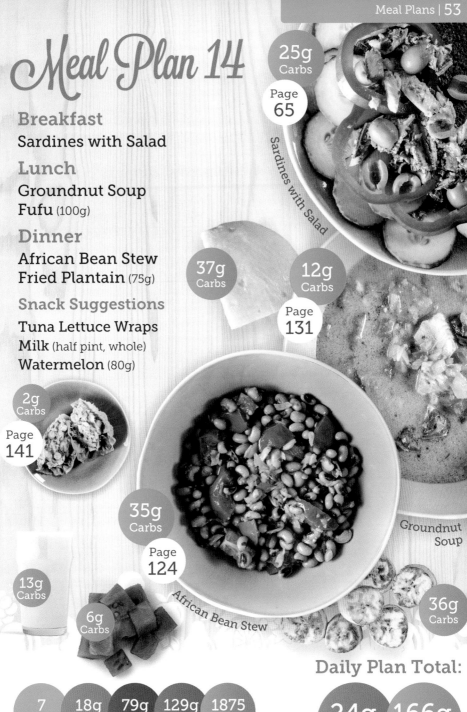

25g Carbs

Page 65

Sardines with Salad

37g Carbs

12g Carbs

Page 131

2g Carbs

Page 141

35g Carbs

Page 124

African Bean Stew

13g Carbs

6g Carbs

36g Carbs

Groundnut Soup

7 5-a-day	18g SatFat	79g Fat	129g Protein	1875 Cals

Daily Plan Total:

24g Fibre

166g Carbs

See page 31 for more info on adding extra carbs

Kale Kerfuffle Smoothie

Get a great green wake-up call
with this apple and veg mix

Ingredients

1	**Green Apple** (small)
½	**Celery** stalk
⅙	**Courgette**
2	handfuls **Kale**
2	sprigs **Parsley**
¼	**Lemon** (juice only)
80ml	Water
6	Ice Cubes

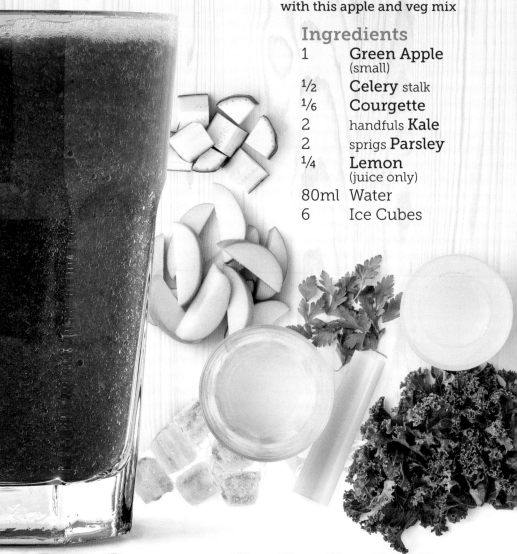

17g Carbs   **6g** Fibre

85 Cals   **3g** Protein   **1g** Fat   **0g** SatFat   **2½** 5-a-day

Weight | 430g

Cauli Smoothie

A surprisingly tasty mix of cauliflower and apple with a hint of aniseed!

Ingredients

½	Red Apple
80g	Cauliflower
1	Carrot
¼	Cucumber
80g	Fennel
2 inch	Ginger (peeled)
½	Lime (juice only)
140ml	Water
6	Ice Cubes

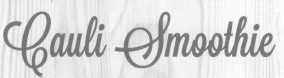

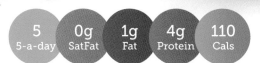

5 5-a-day

0g SatFat

1g Fat

4g Protein

110 Cals

9g Fibre

21g Carbs

Weight | 630g

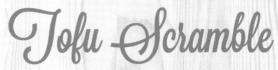

Tofu Scramble

With 13g protein and 2 portions of veg, this light breakfast plate is a great start to the day!

Ingredients

8	**Cherry Tomatoes** (quartered)
1/8	**Green Pepper** (diced)
1/8	**Red Pepper** (diced)
1/3	**Red Onion** (finely chopped)
150g	**Silken Tofu** (crumbled)
1 sprig	**Parsley** (large, chopped)
1	handful **Rocket**

Preparation

1. Dry fry the **tomatoes**, **pepper** and **onion** for 5 mins.
2. Add the **tofu** and heat through.
3. Remove from the heat and stir in the **parsley**.
4. Serve on a bed of **rocket**.

11g Carbs

3g Fibre

135 Cals

13g Protein

5g Fat

1g SatFat

2 5-a-day

Weight | 260g

Rye Bread & Nut Butter

Crispy, crunchy, chunky, yummy...
and ready in minutes!

Ingredients

1 slice **Rye Bread** (toasted)
20g   **Peanut Butter**

Preparation

1. Top the **rye toast** with
   the **peanut butter**.
2. Serve and enjoy!

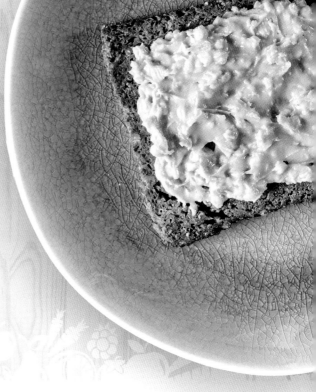

0 5-a-day	2g SatFat	11g Fat	9g Protein	230 Cals

Weight | 70g

4g Fibre	26g Carbs

Cheesy Breakfast Mushroom

Mushroom burger for breakfast? Yes please!
This one is flavoured with garlic and cheese

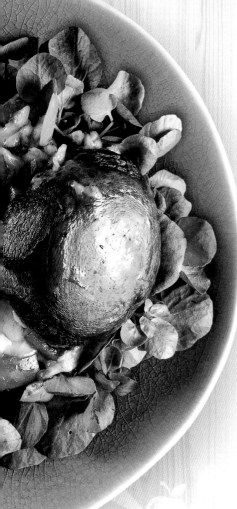

Ingredients

2	**Portobello Mushrooms**
¼	**Red Romano Pepper** (chopped)
1 clove	**Garlic** (minced)
50g	**Smoked Cheddar** (sliced)
1	large handful **Watercress**

Preparation

1. Lay one **mushroom** topside down on a baking tray.
2. Sprinkle with half the **pepper** and half the **garlic**.
3. Lay the sliced **cheese** on top, then the remaining pepper and garlic, to make a stack.
4. Top with the other mushroom and press down gently.
5. Bake for 12 mins at 180°C, turning once.
6. Serve on a bed of **watercress**.

3g Carbs

2g Fibre

250 Cals

18g Protein

18g Fat

11g SatFat

1½ 5-a-day

Weight | 200g

Classic Cooked Breakfast

If you can't resist a fry-up, try this healthy version. It even has 2 of your 5-a-day!

Ingredients

2	**Back Bacon** rashers
80g	**Mushrooms** (sliced)
8	**Cherry Tomatoes** (on the vine)
1	**Egg** (whisked)
1	handful **Spinach**

Preparation

1. Dry fry the **bacon**, **mushrooms** and **tomatoes** for 10 mins.
2. Set aside the mixture on a warm plate, then add the **egg** to the same pan. Stir until scrambled and completely cooked.
3. Serve with fresh **spinach** on the side.

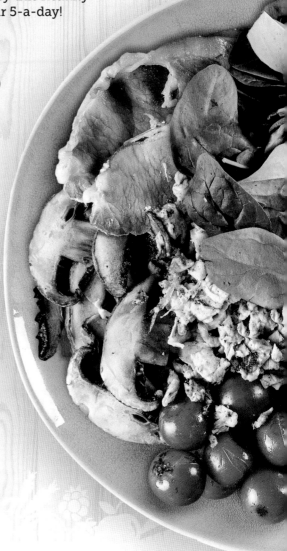

2 5-a-day	5g SatFat	16g Fat	20g Protein	260 Cals	1g Fibre	5g Carbs

Weight | 190g

Egg, Salmon & Asparagus

Start your day a colourful way with this smorgasbord of flavours!

Ingredients

1	**Egg**
50g	**Natural Yogurt**
1 sprig	**Dill** (finely chopped)
¼	**Lemon** (juice only)
75g	**Smoked Salmon**
80g	**Asparagus** (blanched)

Preparation

1. Poach the **egg** in boiling water (with or without vinegar) until the white is completely set and opaque, and the yolk is firm.

2. To make the dressing, mix the **yogurt**, **dill** and **lemon juice**.

3. Serve the **salmon** and **asparagus** topped with the egg and dressing.

6g Carbs

2g Fibre

275 Cals

31g Protein

14g Fat

4g SatFat

1 5-a-day

Weight | 280g

Veggie Breakfast

This vibrant veggie ensemble is loaded with nutrients and 3½ of your 5-a-day

Ingredients

1	**Egg**
80g	**Mushrooms** (sliced)
8	**Cherry Tomatoes** (on the vine)
1 tsp	**Olive Oil**
2	handfuls **Spinach**
½	**Avocado** (sliced)

Preparation

1. Poach the **egg** in boiling water (with or without vinegar) until the white is completely set and opaque, and the yolk is firm.

2. Meanwhile, pan fry the **mushrooms** and **tomatoes** in 1 tsp **oil**, until they start to colour.

3. Add the **spinach** for a couple of minutes, until it starts to wilt.

4. Serve as a stack, with spinach on the bottom, **avocado**, mushroom and topped with the egg.

5. Finally, decorate the plate with the tomatoes and any juices from the pan.

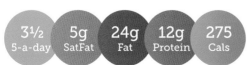

3½ 5-a-day	5g SatFat	24g Fat	12g Protein	275 Cals

Weight | 245g

5g Fibre   **5g** Carbs

Chia Seed Breakfast Pot

This vanilla-infused brekkie provides a third of your daily fibre needs before you've left the house!

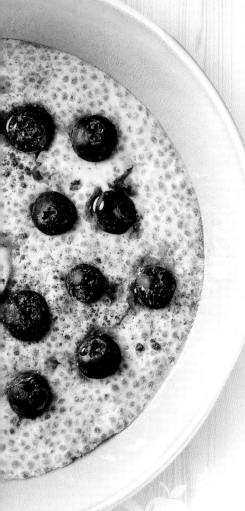

Ingredients

25g	Dark Chia Seeds
180ml	Almond Milk
½	Vanilla Pod (seeds only)
80g	Greek Yogurt
40g	Blueberries
1 tsp	Maple Syrup
pinch	Cinnamon (ground)

Preparation

1. Combine the **chia seeds** with the **almond milk** and **vanilla seeds**.

2. Soak in the fridge for 6 hours, or overnight.

3. Mix the **yogurt** through the chia seed mixture.

4. Top with **blueberries**, **maple syrup** and a pinch of **cinnamon**.

20g Carbs

10g Fibre

290 Cals

11g Protein

17g Fat

5g SatFat

½ 5-a-day

Weight | 335g

Smoked Salmon & Egg

A healthy take on eggs royale. Can't go wrong with the tried and tested egg & salmon combo!

Ingredients

1	**Egg**
1 slice	**Rye Bread**
⅛	**Cucumber** (sliced)
1	handful **Rocket**
50g	**Smoked Salmon** (sliced)
¼	**Lemon** (juice only)
1 sprig	**Dill** (chopped)

Preparation

1. Poach the **egg** in boiling water (with or without vinegar) until the white is completely set and opaque, and the yolk is firm.
2. Toast the **rye bread**, then layer with **cucumber**, **rocket**, **salmon** and egg.
3. Serve drizzled with **lemon juice** and sprinkled with **dill**.

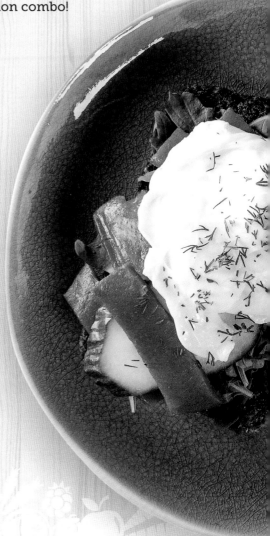

1 5-a-day	3g SatFat	11g Fat	26g Protein	290 Cals	4g Fibre	24g Carbs

Weight | 215g

Avocado & Eggs

This combination of avo & eggs is a great source of good-quality protein & healthy fats

Ingredients

2 **Eggs**
¼ **Lemon** (juice only)
½ **Avocado** (sliced)

Preparation

1. Poach the **eggs** in boiling water (with or without vinegar) until the whites are completely set and opaque, and the yolks are firm.

2. Drizzle the **lemon juice** over the **avocado** and serve with the poached eggs.

2g Carbs

3g Fibre

290 Cals

16g Protein

24g Fat

6g SatFat

1 5-a-day

Weight | 160g

Sardines with Salad

A simple way to pack in the protein at the start of your day. Full-flavoured and quick to make!

Ingredients

1 slice	**Rye Bread**	(toasted)
100g	**Sardines**	(tinned)
1/8	**Cucumber**	(sliced)
1/4	**Red Pepper**	(sliced)
4	**Olives**	(sliced)

Preparation

1. Top the **rye toast** with **sardines**.
2. Serve with **cucumber**, **pepper** and **olives**.

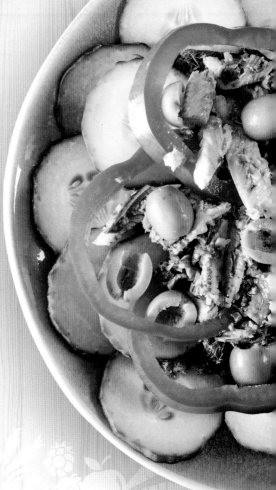

1 5-a-day	3g SatFat	12g Fat	27g Protein	305 Cals

Weight | 235g

5g Fibre	25g Carbs

Oat Khichdi

The dal and oats both offer slow-releasing carbs
in this deliciously colourful dish

Ingredients

30g	dried **Yellow Mung Dal**
½ tsp	**Cumin Seeds**
1 tbsp	**Olive Oil**
1 inch	**Ginger** (grated)
pinch	**Asafoetida**
½	**Carrot** (diced)
40g	**Cauliflower** (chopped)
⅛	**Onion** (diced)
40g	**Peas**
¼	**Red Pepper** (chopped)
pinch	**Turmeric** (ground)
2 tbsp	**Jumbo Oats**

Preparation

1. Cook the **mung dal** according to packet instructions. Drain and set aside.
2. Fry the **cumin seeds** in 1 tbsp **oil**. When they sizzle add the **ginger** and **asafoetida**.
3. Add **all the vegetables** and sauté for 2 mins.
4. Stir in the dal and **turmeric**. Fry for a further 2 mins.
5. Pour in the **oats** and 250ml water. Bring to the boil.
6. Simmer for 5 mins, or until the sauce thickens, then serve.

40g Carbs

12g Fibre

335 Cals

13g Protein

15g Fat

2g SatFat

2½ 5-a-day

Weight | 450g

Mushroom Pepper Omelette

Short on time? Whip up a mouth-watering cheesy omelette in minutes!

Ingredients

40g	**Mushrooms** (thinly sliced)
¼	**Red Pepper** (thinly sliced)
2 tsp	**Olive Oil**
1	handful **Spinach**
2	**Eggs** (whisked)
8	**Cherry Tomatoes** (on the vine)
20g	**Cheddar Cheese** (grated)
1 sprig	**Parsley** (chopped)

Preparation

1. Pan fry the **mushrooms** and **pepper** in 2 tsp **oil**, until soft.

2. Add the **spinach** and cook for a further minute.

3. Pour the **eggs** over the vegetables in the pan.

4. When the egg mixture starts to firm up, drop in the **cherry tomatoes** to cook at the side of the pan.

5. Sprinkle the **cheese** and **parsley** on top. Heat for a further 2 mins (or until the eggs are completely cooked), then serve.

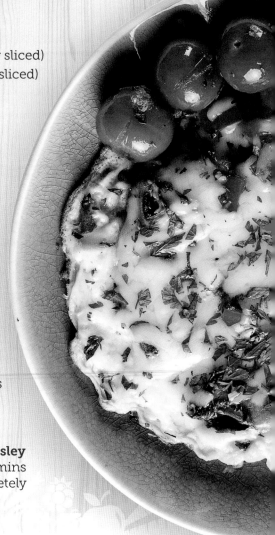

2 5-a-day	9g SatFat	27g Fat	22g Protein	375 Cals	2g Fibre	6g Carbs

Weight | 310g

Yogurt, Nuts & Blueberries

A medley of textures... creamy yogurt, crunchy nuts & seeds, and juicy blueberry bombs

Ingredients

2 tbsp **Pecans** (chopped)
2 tbsp **Mixed Seeds**
pinch **Cinnamon** (ground)
200g **Natural Yogurt**
40g **Blueberries**

Preparation

1. In a dry pan over a medium heat, toast the **pecans** and **seeds** with **cinnamon** until aromatic.

2. Spoon the **yogurt** into a bowl, and serve topped with the toasted nuts and **blueberries**.

17g Carbs

5g Fibre

410 Cals

15g Protein

31g Fat

7g SatFat

½ 5-a-day

Weight | 270g

Eggs & Fried Plantain

Sweet golden plantain is the perfect partner for scrambled eggs in this delectable jumble

Ingredients

120g	**Plantain**	(thickly sliced)
1 tbsp	**Rapeseed Oil**	
¼	**Red Pepper**	(sliced)
4	**Cherry Tomatoes** (halved)	
2	**Eggs**	(whisked)

Preparation

1. Fry the **plantain** slices in ½ tbsp **oil** for 5 mins, until golden on both sides. Set aside.

2. In the same pan, sauté the **pepper** and **tomatoes** in ½ tbsp oil for 4 mins. Set aside.

3. Add the **eggs** to the pan and stir on a gentle heat for 2 mins, until scrambled and completely cooked.

4. Serve the scrambled egg over the pepper, and top with the plantain and tomatoes.

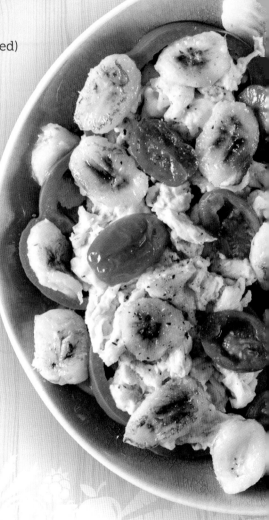

2 5-a-day	4g SatFat	23g Fat	17g Protein	425 Cals

3g Fibre	38g Carbs

Weight | 270g

Fruity Porridge

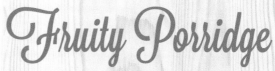

Stay full all morning with this tasty
bowl of slow-releasing carbs

Ingredients

6 tbsp	**Jumbo Oats**
200ml	**Milk** (whole)
¼	**Apple** (grated)
2 tbsp	**Pecans**
40g	**Blueberries**
1 tbsp	**Natural Yogurt**

Preparation

1. Heat the **oats** with the **milk**, grated **apple** and 75ml water. Bring to the boil.

2. Turn down the heat and simmer for 10 mins, or until the oats are cooked.

3. Serve scattered with **pecans**, **blueberries** and a tablespoon of **yogurt**.

41g Carbs

5g Fibre

425 Cals

13g Protein

24g Fat

7g SatFat

1 5-a-day

Weight | 280g

Chicken Congee Soup

Loaded with flavour, this chicken rice soup puts a smile on your face every time!

Ingredients

400ml	**Chicken Stock** (½ cube)
½ inch	**Ginger** (sliced)
35g	uncooked **Basmati Rice**
150g	**Chicken Breast** (raw, diced)
½ tsp	**Chinese Rice Wine**
⅛	**Onion** (thinly sliced)
1 clove	**Garlic** (sliced)
1 tbsp	**Rapeseed Oil**
1	**Spring Onion** (sliced)
½ tsp	**Sesame Oil**
½ tsp	**Soy Sauce**

Preparation

1. Boil the **stock** with the **ginger**. Reduce the heat, add the **rice**, cover and simmer for 20 mins, or until almost all of the water has been absorbed.

2. Stir in the **chicken** and heat for 5 mins (or until the chicken is completely cooked). Add the **rice wine** and remove from heat.

3. In a separate pan, fry the **onion** and **garlic** in 1 tbsp **rapeseed oil** on a medium-high heat for 5 mins or until crispy. Keep moving to avoid burning.

4. Serve the soup topped with the fried garlic and onion, sliced **spring onion**, **sesame oil** and the **soy sauce**.

½ 5-a-day	2g SatFat	16g Fat	40g Protein	435 Cals	1g Fibre	33g Carbs

Weight | 355g

Cornmeal Porridge

Sweet, spiced and a little bit nutty, this creamy porridge
won't let you down on a chilly morning!

Ingredients

300ml	**Soya Milk** (unsweetened)
40g	**Cornmeal** (sieved)
2	**Cloves**
pinch	**Cinnamon** (ground)
pinch	**Nutmeg**
2 drops	**Vanilla Extract**
1 tsp	**Honey**
1 tbsp	**Brazil Nuts** (chopped)
2 tbsp	**Cashews** (chopped)

Preparation

1. Warm the **soya milk** on a medium heat and bring to a gentle simmer.
2. Stir in the **cornmeal**, **cloves**, **cinnamon** and **nutmeg**.
3. Whisk the mixture until it starts to thicken.
4. Drizzle in the **vanilla extract** and **honey**.
5. Remove the cloves, then serve topped with the **nuts** and a pinch of salt. Enjoy!

42g Carbs

4g Fibre

445 Cals

16g Protein

23g Fat

5g SatFat

0 5-a-day

Weight | 320g

Ackee & Saltfish

This classic Jamaican dish is high in protein and boasts 3 of your 5-a-day. Tuck in!

Ingredients

100g	dried **Saltfish**
½	**Onion** (sliced)
pinch	**Thyme** (dried)
1	**Tomato** (chopped)
¼	**Red Pepper** (chopped)
1 tsp	**Tomato Purée**
1 tbsp	**Olive Oil**
100g	**Ackee** (tinned)

Preparation

1. Soak the **saltfish** for 24 hours before use, changing the water several times.

2. Boil the fish for 20 mins. Drain, then break into small pieces.

3. Fry the **onion**, **thyme**, **tomato**, **pepper** and **tomato purée** in 1 tbsp **oil** for 5 mins.

4. Stir in the fish and heat for 2 mins.

5. Add the drained **ackee**. Resist stirring, to keep the ackee whole. Leave for 1 min to allow the ackee to warm through.

6. Serve with fried plantain (optional, see page 208) and sprinkled with black pepper.

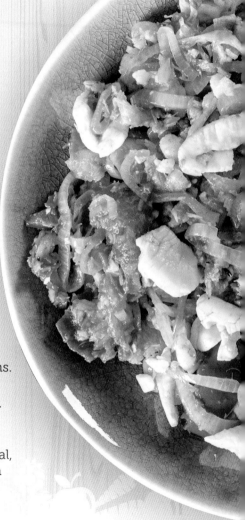

3 5-a-day	2g SatFat	29g Fat	39g Protein	455 Cals	4g Fibre	11g Carbs

Weight | 375g

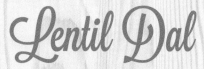

Lentil Dal

Chana dal provides the slow-releasing carbs
in this classic, colourful vegan curry

Ingredients

40g	dried **Chana Dal** (soaked)
½ tsp	**Cumin Seeds**
¼ tsp	**Garam Masala**
½ tsp	**Mustard Seeds**
½ tsp	**Turmeric** (ground)
2	**Curry Leaves**
1 tsp	**Olive Oil**
¼	**Onion** (diced)
½	**Green Chilli** (diced)
1 clove	**Garlic** (minced)
80g	**Tomato** (chopped)
1 sprig	**Coriander** (large, chopped)

Preparation

1. Rinse the pre-soaked **dal** and place
   in a pan with 200ml water. Bring to
   the boil and simmer for 40 mins, or
   until soft. Drain and discard water.

2. Fry the **spices** and **curry leaves** in
   1 tsp **oil**, allowing the seeds to sizzle
   and pop for a minute or two.

3. Stir in the **onion**, **chilli** and
   garlic. Cook for 3 mins.

4. Add the dal, **tomato** and 100ml
   water. Bring to the boil and simmer
   until the dal reduces and thickens.
   Add more water if too thick.

5. Serve with fresh **coriander**.

32g Carbs
8g Fibre

215 Cals
11g Protein
6g Fat
1g SatFat
2 5-a-day

Weight | 240g

Paneer Masala

Ingredients

1	Bay Leaf
1	Clove
1 stick	Cinnamon
½	Red Chilli (sliced)
1 tsp	Coriander Seeds (crushed)
2 tsp	Butter
1 tsp	Olive Oil
¼	Onion (sliced)
1 inch	Ginger (grated)
1 clove	Garlic (minced)
pinch	Coriander (ground)
pinch	Chilli Powder
40g	Tomato (chopped)
50g	Paneer (cubed)
¼	Yellow Pepper (chopped)
80g	Petit Pois
25g	Natural Yogurt
pinch	Fenugreek Seeds

Preparation

1. Sauté the **bay leaf, clove, cinnamon stick, red chilli** and half the **coriander seeds** in 1 tsp **butter** and 1 tsp **oil** for 1 min.

2. Stir in the **onion, ginger** and **garlic**, before adding the **ground coriander, chilli powder** and **tomato**. Fry for 5 mins, remove the cinnamon stick, add 50ml water and purée.

3. Sauté the **paneer** and **pepper** in 1 tsp butter for 1 min. Add the **peas**, puréed mixture and 150ml water. Bubble on a high heat until the sauce has reduced.

4. Remove from the heat, stirring in the **yogurt** and **fenugreek seeds**. Sprinkle with the remaining coriander seeds and serve.

2½ 5-a-day	13g SatFat	25g Fat	21g Protein	380 Cals		7g Fibre	18g Carbs

Weight | 325g

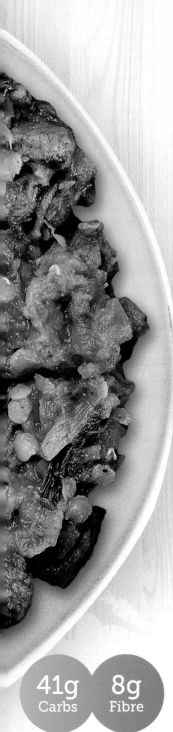

Lamb Dhansak

Like lamb? You'll love this hearty bowlful!

Ingredients

70g	Stewing Lamb (raw, diced)
1 pod	Cardamom (seeds only, ground)
pinch	Coriander (ground)
pinch	Cumin (ground)
pinch	Turmeric (ground)
¼	Onion (diced)
1 inch	Ginger (grated)
1 clove	Garlic (minced)
½	Red Chilli (sliced)
150g	Chopped Tomatoes (tinned)
80g	Butternut Squash (cubed)
40g	dried Red Split Lentils
200ml	Beef Stock (½ cube)
2	handfuls Spinach
1 sprig	Coriander (large, chopped)

Preparation

1. Coat the **lamb** in the **dry spices** and dry fry until browned and aromatic.

2. Add the **onion** and fry for 5 mins until soft.

3. Stir in the **ginger**, **garlic** and sliced **chilli** and cook for a further 2 mins.

4. Mix through the **tomatoes**, **squash**, **lentils** and **stock**, and bring to the boil.

5. Simmer for 25 mins, or until the lentils and lamb are cooked and the curry is thick.

6. Fold in the **spinach** and allow to wilt. Serve topped with the fresh **coriander**.

41g Carbs

8g Fibre

390 Cals

33g Protein

12g Fat

5g SatFat

3½ 5-a-day

Weight | 410g

Sweet Potato Curry

A full-flavoured veggie delight to tickle your taste buds in all the right places!

Ingredients

⅓	**Red Onion** (thinly sliced)
1 tsp	**Olive Oil**
1 tbsp	**Coconut Cream**
1 tbsp	**Curry Paste**
80g	**Cauliflower** (small florets)
1	**Red Chilli** (sliced)
1 inch	**Ginger** (grated)
80g	**Sweet Potato** (cubed)
80g	**Chickpeas** (tinned)
150ml	**Vegetable Stock** (½ cube)
80g	**Tomato** (chopped)
1 sprig	**Coriander** (large, chopped)

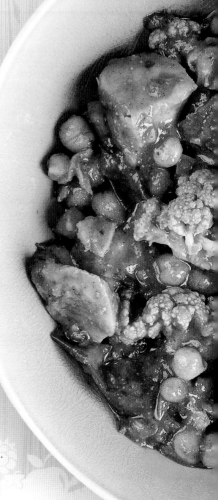

Preparation

1. Fry the **onion** in 1 tsp **oil** until soft. Stir in the **coconut cream** and **curry paste**.

2. Add the **cauliflower, chilli, ginger, sweet potato** and **chickpeas**. Cook for 5 mins.

3. Pour in the **stock**, along with the **tomato** and half of the **coriander**.

4. Bring to the boil, then simmer for 20 mins, or until the potato is cooked.

5. Serve sprinkled with the remaining coriander.

3½ 5-a-day	10g SatFat	21g Fat	12g Protein	395 Cals

11g Fibre	43g Carbs

Weight | 620g

Okra & Lentil Curry

Oh my goodness... this nutritious curry has
4 of your 5-a-day and 50% of your daily fibre!

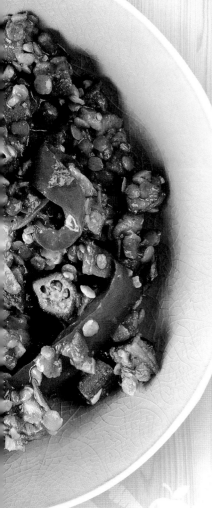

Ingredients

160g	**Aubergine** (cubed)
½	**Red Pepper** (sliced)
1 tbsp	**Olive Oil**
¼	**Onion** (sliced)
¼ tsp	**Black Mustard Seeds**
1 clove	**Garlic** (minced)
1 tsp	**Curry Paste**
80g	**Okra** (chopped)
60g	dried **Red Split Lentils**
300ml	**Vegetable Stock** (½ cube)
1 sprig	**Coriander** (large, chopped)

Preparation

1. Mix the **aubergine** and **pepper** with ½ tbsp **oil** and bake at 180°C for 25 mins.

2. Meanwhile, fry the **onion** in ½ tbsp oil until soft, then add the **mustard seeds**, **garlic**, **curry paste** and **okra**.

3. Stir in the **lentils** and **stock**. Bring to the boil, then simmer for 20 mins or until the lentils are cooked.

4. Fold in the roasted veggies, top with **coriander**, and serve.

48g Carbs

16g Fibre

400 Cals

20g Protein

16g Fat

2g SatFat

4 5-a-day

Weight | 500g

Jamaican Chicken Curry

The ultimate curry... with 4 of your 5-a-day, a whopping 48g protein, and nearly half your daily fibre needs!

Ingredients

1 tsp	**Curry Powder**
1 tbsp	**Olive Oil**
150g	**Chicken Breast** (raw, skinless, cubed)
1/3	**Red Onion** (thinly sliced)
1/2	**Red Chilli** (chopped)
120g	**Tomato** (chopped)
1/4	**Red Pepper** (sliced)
1/4	**Yellow Pepper** (sliced)
80g	**Natural Yogurt**
100ml	**Chicken Stock** (½ cube)
80g	**Kidney Beans** (tinned)
1/4	**Mango** (cubed)
1 sprig	**Coriander** (chopped)

Preparation

1. Coat the chicken in **curry powder**. Heat 1 tbsp **oil** in a pan, add the **chicken** and brown for 3 mins.

2. Stir in the **onion**, **chilli**, **tomato** and **peppers**. Fry for a further 5 mins.

3. Pour in the **yogurt** and **stock**. Bring to the boil, then simmer until the chicken is thoroughly cooked.

4. Add the **beans** and **mango**. Cook gently to warm the beans.

5. Sprinkle with chopped **coriander** to serve.

| 4 5-a-day | 4g SatFat | 18g Fat | 48g Protein | 485 Cals | 14g Fibre | 35g Carbs |

Weight | 540g

Coconut Fish Curry

There's something special about a fish and coconut combo - a marriage made in heaven!

Ingredients

½ tsp	Cumin Seeds
1 tbsp	Olive Oil
1 tsp	Butter
¼	Onion (diced)
pinch	Chilli Powder (mild)
pinch	Garam Masala
pinch	Turmeric (ground)
120g	Tomato (chopped)
½	Green Chilli (sliced)
150ml	Coconut Milk (tinned)
140g	Cod (fillet, chunks, sustainable)
1 sprig	Coriander (large, chopped)

Preparation

1. Gently fry the **cumin seeds** in the **oil** and **butter** for 1 min, or until aromatic. Add the **onions** and fry until golden.

2. Stir in the remaining **spices** with the **tomato** and **chilli**. Cook until the tomato has broken down.

3. Pour in the **coconut milk** and bring to the boil.

4. Add the **cod**, reduce the heat, cover and simmer for 5 mins, or until the fish is completely cooked.

5. Sprinkle with **coriander** and serve.

14g Carbs

3g Fibre

550 Cals

28g Protein

43g Fat

27g SatFat

1½ 5-a-day

Weight | 360g

Lamb & Spinach Stew

Is it a stew? Is it a curry? Dig in and find out.
Comes with a bonus of 49g protein!

Ingredients

1 inch	**Ginger** (grated)
2 cloves	**Garlic** (minced)
1 tsp	**Coriander Seeds**
150g	**Stewing Lamb** (raw, lean, diced)
½	**Onion** (thinly sliced)
2 tsp	**Rapeseed Oil**
½ tsp	**Turmeric** (ground)
½	**Red Chilli** (diced)
100g	**Natural Yogurt**
3	handfuls **Spinach**

Preparation

1. Using a pestle & mortar, crush the **ginger**, **garlic**, and **coriander seeds** to a paste, with a pinch of salt. Coat the **lamb** with the paste and leave to marinate for 1 hour minimum.

2. Fry the **onions** in 2 tsp **oil** until golden. Remove ¼ of the onions and set aside.

3. Add the lamb, **turmeric**, and **chilli** to the pan with the remaining onions. Sauté on a high heat for 3 mins, to seal the meat. Reduce the heat, cover with a lid and cook gently for 2 hours.

4. Gradually stir in the **yogurt**, until fully combined.

5. Mix through the **spinach** and simmer for 5 mins, or until the sauce has thickened. Serve with the onions.

2 5-a-day	12g SatFat	34g Fat	49g Protein	570 Cals	4g Fibre	18g Carbs

Weight | 345g

Spinach Stew & Rice

Light & nutritious, this simple stew contains half of your 5-a-day

Ingredients

35g	uncooked **Brown Basmati Rice**
¼	**Onion** (chopped)
1 clove	**Garlic** (minced)
1 tsp	**Rapeseed Oil**
pinch	**Cayenne Pepper**
1 tsp	**Curry Powder**
pinch	**Black Pepper** (ground)
80g	**Tomatoes** (chopped)
4	handfuls **Spinach**

Preparation

1. Cook the **rice** according to the packet instructions.
2. Fry the **onion** and **garlic** in 1 tsp **oil** for 5 mins, until softened.
3. Add the **cayenne pepper**, **curry powder** and **black pepper**. Sauté for 2 mins, stirring continuously.
4. Mix in the **tomatoes** and 200ml water. Cover and simmer for 10 mins.
5. Add the **spinach**, cover and cook on a low heat for a further 15 mins, or until the stew thickens.
6. Serve on the cooked basmati rice.

35g Carbs · **6g** Fibre

215 Cals · **6g** Protein · **6g** Fat · **1g** SatFat · **2½** 5-a-day

Weight | 275g

Quinoa Stuffed Mushrooms

The quinoa in this dish is a great source of plant-based protein

Ingredients

1/3	**Red Onion** (finely chopped)
1 tsp	**Olive Oil**
50g	**Ricotta**
80g	cooked **Quinoa**
1 sprig	**Parsley** (large, chopped)
1/2 tsp	**Oregano** (dried)
2	**Portobello Mushrooms**
8	**Cherry Tomatoes** (on the vine)
1	large handful **Watercress**

Preparation

1. Fry the **onion** in 1 tsp **oil** until soft.

2. Mix the onion with the **ricotta**, cooked **quinoa**, **herbs**, salt and pepper.

3. Stuff the **mushrooms** with the ricotta mixture and roast, along with the **tomatoes** (on the vine), for 20 mins at 200°C.

4. Serve on a bed of **watercress**.

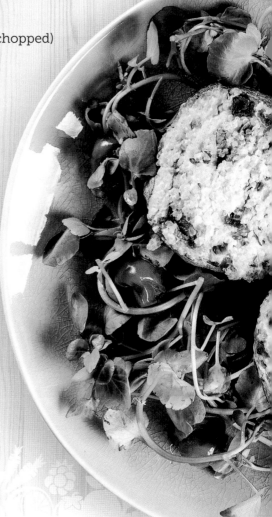

2½ 5-a-day	4g SatFat	13g Fat	13g Protein	265 Cals	7g Fibre	24g Carbs

Weight | 330g

Cauliflower Risotto

Slurp up this soupy, riceless risotto - around half the calories of normal risotto!

Ingredients

¼	Onion (sliced)
1 tsp	Olive Oil
80g	Mushrooms (sliced)
1 clove	Garlic (minced)
160g	Cauliflower (grated)
150ml	Vegetable Stock (½ cube)
40g	Petit Pois
1 sprig	Thyme (leaves, chopped)
1 sprig	Rosemary (leaves, chopped)
40g	Greek Yogurt
20g	Parmesan (grated)

Preparation

1. Fry the **onion** in 1 tsp **oil** for 1 min on a medium heat. Add the **mushrooms** and cook for 4 mins.
2. Next, stir in the **garlic** and **cauliflower**. Fry for 2 mins, then add the **stock** and **peas**.
3. Bring to the boil and simmer for 5 mins.
4. Sprinkle in the **thyme** and **rosemary**, and cook for 1 min, stirring in the **yogurt** and **parmesan**.
5. Remove from the heat and serve.

17g Carbs	7g Fibre

265 Cals	17g Protein	15g Fat	7g SatFat	3 5-a-day

Weight | 330g

Baked Aubergine & Feta

An easy way to bagsie half of your 5-a-day!

Ingredients

40g	uncooked **Bulgur Wheat**
1/2	**Aubergine**
8	**Cherry Tomatoes** (halved)
25g	**Feta** (cubed)
1 sprig	**Rosemary** (leaves, chopped)
1 sprig	**Oregano** (chopped)
1 sprig	**Basil** (chopped)
8	**Olives** (chopped)
1 clove	**Garlic** (sliced)

Preparation

1. Cook the **bulgur wheat** according to the packet instructions and set aside.

2. Bake the **aubergine** at 200°C for 10 mins.

3. Meanwhile, mix the bulgur wheat with the **tomatoes**, **feta**, **herbs** and **olives**.

4. Spoon ¾ of the mixture onto the aubergine, add the **garlic** and continue to roast for 20 mins, or until the aubergine is cooked.

5. Serve with the remaining bulgur wheat mixture on the side.

2½ 5-a-day	4g SatFat	9g Fat	10g Protein	265 Cals	7g Fibre	37g Carbs

Weight | 325g

Pollock & Chickpeas

Pollock packs a protein punch in this winning combination

Ingredients

140g	**Pollock** (raw fillet)
¼	**Lemon** (juice only)
8	**Cherry Tomatoes**
1 tsp	**Olive Oil**
80g	**Chickpeas** (tinned)
pinch	**Sumac** (large)
4	handfuls **Spinach**

Preparation

1. Season the **fish** with **lemon juice**, salt & pepper. Place on a baking tray, surrounded by the **tomatoes**.

2. Bake for 12 mins at 200°C, or until the fish is thoroughly cooked.

3. Meanwhile, heat 1 tsp **oil** in a pan. Add the **chickpeas** and **sumac**, frying for 3 mins.

4. Drop in the **spinach** and cook for a further 2 mins.

5. Serve the fish on top of the chickpeas, spinach and tomatoes, drizzling any pan juices over the top.

17g Carbs

8g Fibre

270 Cals

32g Protein

9g Fat

1g SatFat

4 5-a-day

Weight | 305g

Moroccan Veg & Chickpeas

A spicy concoction, delivering a massive 7½ portions of veg and over half your daily fibre requirements. Tuck in!

Ingredients

80g	**Aubergine** (cubed)
½	**Beetroot** (raw, cubed)
½	**Carrot** (chopped)
80g	**Cauliflower** (florets, halved)
⅓	**Courgette** (cubed)
⅓	**Red Onion** (wedges)
¼	**Red Pepper** (chopped)
¼	**Yellow Pepper** (chopped)
2 cloves	**Garlic** (in skin)
2 tsp	**Olive Oil**
pinch	**Chilli Flakes, Coriander Seeds, Cumin Seeds, Nigella Seeds & Sumac**
4	**Cherry Tomatoes**
100g	**Chickpeas** (tinned)
1	handful **Kale**
5	**Mint** leaves (torn)
1 sprig	**Coriander** (large, chopped)

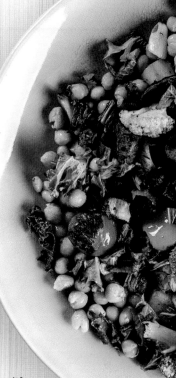

Preparation

1. Mix the **veg** (except the tomatoes and kale) with 1 tsp **oil**, **garlic** and **spices**. Bake at 200°C for 20 mins.
2. When cooked, squeeze the roasted garlic out of its skin and fry with the **tomatoes** in 1 tsp oil for 1 min.
3. Add 100ml water, bring to the boil, simmer until reduced.
4. Stir in the **chickpeas**, adding the **kale** after 1 min.
5. Plate up the roasted veg surrounded by the chickpea mixture, and scatter with **mint** and **coriander** to serve.

7½ 5-a-day	2g SatFat	13g Fat	15g Protein	325 Cals	18g Fibre	39g Carbs

Weight | 415g

Prawn & Kale Stir-fry

A vibrant Asian taste sensation
that is ready in minutes

Ingredients

1 tsp	Olive Oil
100g	cooked King Prawns
½	Red Pepper (sliced)
½	Red Chilli (finely chopped)
1 clove	Garlic (minced)
1 inch	Ginger (finely chopped)
80g	cooked Soya Beans
2 tsp	Soy Sauce
2 tsp	Fish Sauce
2 tsp	Mirin
80g	Beansprouts
2	handfuls Kale
1 sprig	Coriander (chopped)
½	Lime (juice only)

Preparation

1. Heat 1 tsp **oil** in a wok until very hot. Fry the **prawns**, **pepper**, **chilli**, **garlic** and **ginger** for 2 mins.

2. Add the **soya beans**, **soy sauce**, **fish sauce** and **mirin**, and heat for another minute.

3. Sprinkle in the **beansprouts** and **kale**, cooking for a further 2 mins (or until the prawns are completely cooked).

4. Serve scattered with **coriander** and a squeeze of **lime**.

20g Carbs

9g Fibre

325 Cals

32g Protein

11g Fat

1g SatFat

3½ 5-a-day

Weight | 280g

Beef & Mushroom Stir-fry

This speedy stir-fry provides 4 of your
5-a-day in record time!

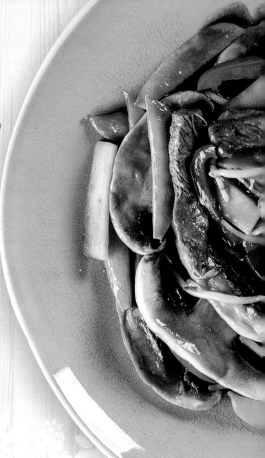

Ingredients

1 tsp	Olive Oil
100g	Beef Sirloin (raw, thin strips)
1 inch	Ginger (finely sliced)
1 clove	Garlic (minced)
40g	Bamboo Shoots
40g	Beansprouts
80g	Mushrooms (sliced)
½	Red Pepper (sliced)
80g	Sugar Snap Peas
2 tbsp	Oyster Sauce
1 tsp	Soy Sauce

Preparation

1. Heat a wok until very hot.
   Add 1 tsp **oil** and the **beef**
   strips, cooking for 3 mins.

2. Add the **ginger, garlic**
   and **all of the vegetables**.
   Fry for a further 2 mins.

3. Stir in the **oyster sauce**
   and **soy sauce**. Cook for
   1 min (or until the beef
   is thoroughly cooked).

4. Serve & enjoy!

4 5-a-day	6g SatFat	18g Fat	29g Protein	330 Cals

Weight | 350g

6g Fibre	16g Carbs

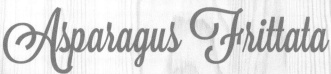

Asparagus Frittata

This satisfying lunch can be eaten hot or cold,
making it perfect for taking to work

Ingredients

¼	**Onion** (sliced)
1 tsp	**Olive Oil**
80g	**Asparagus Tips** (chopped)
20g	**Sun-dried Tomatoes** (chopped)
1 sprig	**Parsley** (large, chopped)
3	**Eggs** (whisked)

Preparation

1. Using a small oven-proof frying pan, gently fry the **onion** for 3 mins in 1 tsp **oil**.
2. Add the **asparagus**, **tomatoes** and **parsley**, and cook for 2 mins to soften.
3. Turn the heat up until the pan sizzles, then add the **eggs** and cook for 2 mins.
4. Place the pan in the oven at 200°C for a further 8 mins, until the frittata is completely set, then serve.

6g Carbs **4g** Fibre

340 Cals **26g** Protein **23g** Fat **5g** SatFat **1½** 5-a-day

Weight | 240g

Jerk Chicken

This finger-licking Caribbean classic offers a whopping 49g protein. Dig in!

Ingredients

pinch	**Allspice** (ground)
pinch	**Black Pepper** (ground)
1 tbsp	**Dark Soy Sauce**
1 inch	**Ginger**
½	**Green Chilli**
pinch	**Nutmeg**
⅛	**Onion**
3 sprigs	**Thyme**
2 tbsp	**Water**
200g	**Chicken Breast** (raw fillet, skinless)
1 tbsp	**Rapeseed Oil**

Preparation

1. Add **all the ingredients**, except the chicken and oil, to a food processor and blitz until smooth.

2. Smother the **chicken** in the marinade sauce and leave in the fridge for at least 30 mins (ideally overnight).

3. After marinating, fry the chicken in 1 tbsp **oil** for 5 mins on each side (until thoroughly cooked), basting with the sauce.

4. Serve with rice & peas (optional, see page 179).

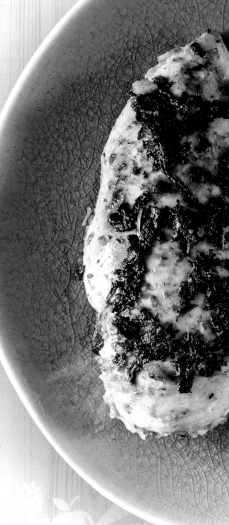

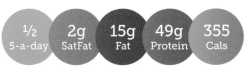

| ½ 5-a-day | 2g SatFat | 15g Fat | 49g Protein | 355 Cals | | 1g Fibre | 7g Carbs |

Weight | 200g

Turkey Mushroom Linguine

If you are short on time, this effortless dish has just 5 ingredients but a whole lot of flavour!

Ingredients

- 40g uncooked **Linguine or Wholemeal Spaghetti**
- 100g **Turkey Breast** (raw, sliced)
- 80g **Chestnut Mushrooms** (sliced)
- 1 tsp **Oregano** (dried)
- 2 tsp **Rapeseed Oil**
- 10g **Parmesan** (grated)

Preparation

1. Cook the **pasta** according to the packet instructions.
2. Meanwhile, fry the **turkey**, **mushrooms** and **oregano** in 2 tsp **oil** for 6 mins, or until the turkey is completely cooked.
3. Combine the mixture with the pasta, stir through the **parmesan** and serve.

28g Carbs

5g Fibre

355 Cals

34g Protein

13g Fat

3g SatFat

1 5-a-day

Weight | 200g

Tuna & Roasted Veg

Get all 5 of your 5-a-day (and 41g protein!) with this succulent tuna steak on a colourful bed of veg

Ingredients

80g	**Aubergine** (cubed)
160g	**Butternut Squash** (cubed)
1/3	**Courgette** (cubed)
2 cloves	**Garlic** (in skin)
pinch	**Oregano** (dried)
1/2	**Red Pepper** (cubed)
1 sprig	**Rosemary** (leaves, chopped)
1/2	**Yellow Pepper** (cubed)
2 tsp	**Olive Oil**
140g	**Tuna Steak** (fresh)
1 tsp	**Cajun Seasoning**
1/2	**Lime** (juice only)

Preparation

1. Combine **all the ingredients** (except the tuna, lime juice, Cajun seasoning and half the oil) and roast at 200°C for 20 mins.

2. Meanwhile, season the **tuna** on each side with the **Cajun seasoning**.

3. Fry the tuna in the remaining 1 tsp **oil** for 2 mins on each side, or until thoroughly cooked. Towards the end, drizzle the **lime juice** over the tuna.

4. When the vegetables are cooked, squeeze the garlic out of its skin.

5. Serve the tuna on the veg, drizzled with pan juices.

5 5-a-day	2g SatFat	10g Fat	41g Protein	355 Cals	11g Fibre	26g Carbs

Weight | 445g

Chickpea Patties

Keep your energy flowing smoothly with the slow-release carbs in these pleasant patties

Ingredients

80g	**Chickpeas** (tinned)
1 clove	**Garlic**
1/3	**Courgette**
1 sprig	**Coriander**
pinch	**Cumin** (ground)
1	**Egg**
2 tbsp	**Oats**
1 tsp	**Olive Oil**
8	**Cherry Tomatoes**
1	handful **Spinach**
1/4	**Avocado** (sliced)

Preparation

1. Blitz the **chickpeas, garlic, courgette, coriander, cumin, egg** and **oats** in a food processor.

2. Use the mixture to form patties, then chill for 1 hour, until firm.

3. Fry the patties in 1 tsp **oil** on a low heat, until crisp on both sides. Set aside on a warm plate.

4. In the same pan, cook the **tomatoes** until they start to burst.

5. To serve, layer the **spinach** and patties, topped with sliced **avocado** and tomatoes.

26g Carbs

10g Fibre

355 Cals

18g Protein

20g Fat

4g SatFat

3½ 5-a-day

Weight | 340g

Turkey Meatballs

An interesting, lighter alternative to a traditional roast dinner

Ingredients

1/8	Onion
1 clove	Garlic
6	Basil leaves
1 sprig	Thyme (leaves)
1	Egg
1	handful Rocket
100g	Turkey Mince (raw)
80g	Sweet Potato (cubed)
1 tsp	Olive Oil
1 sprig	Rosemary (leaves, chopped)
8	Cherry Tomatoes
120g	Green Beans

Preparation

1. Whizz the **onion, garlic, basil, thyme, egg** and **rocket** in a food processor and transfer to a bowl.

2. Use your hands to combine the **mince** with the herb mixture and form into small balls.

3. On a baking tray, coat the **sweet potato** with 1 tsp **oil** and sprinkle with **rosemary**.

4. Place the meatballs on the same tray and cook at 200°C for 20 mins.

5. Add the **tomatoes** to the tray and roast for a further 8 mins, or until the meatballs are thoroughly cooked.

6. Meanwhile, boil or steam the **beans** for 3 mins. Assemble on a plate and enjoy!

2½ 5-a-day	3g SatFat	12g Fat	36g Protein	355 Cals		9g Fibre	26g Carbs

Weight | 280g

Tofu & Bean Stir-fry

The chilli bean sauce offers a full-flavoured jumble for veggie lovers

Ingredients

1 tsp	Olive Oil
1	Carrot (sliced)
160g	Cauliflower (chopped)
⅓	Courgette (batons)
⅓	Red Onion (sliced)
100g	Smoked Tofu (cubed)
1 clove	Garlic (finely sliced)
1 tbsp	Chilli Bean Sauce
1 tsp	Soy Sauce

Preparation

1. Heat a wok until very hot. Add 1 tsp **oil** and **all the vegetables**, frying for 3 mins.
2. Next, mix in the **tofu**, **garlic**, **chilli bean sauce**, **soy sauce** and 2 tbsp water.
3. Cook for a further 2 mins and serve.

24g Carbs

8g Fibre

355 Cals

27g Protein

17g Fat

3g SatFat

3½ 5-a-day

Weight | 300g

Plantain & Beans

A colourful combo to fire up your taste buds
and deliver 3 of your 5-a-day

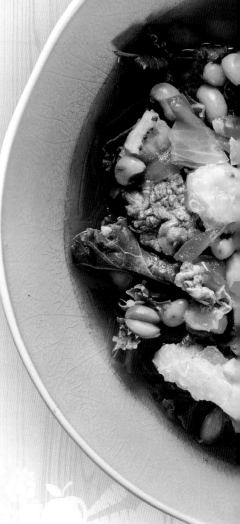

Ingredients

100g	**Beef Sirloin** (raw, lean, chunks)
½ tsp	**Smoked Paprika**
pinch	**Cayenne Pepper**
400ml	**Chicken Stock** (½ cube)
⅛	**Onion** (chopped)
¼	**Red Pepper** (sliced)
¼	**Habanero Chilli** (diced)
80g	**Plantain** (sliced)
80g	**Black Eye Beans** (tinned)
1	handful **Kale**

Preparation

1. Coat the **beef** in **paprika** and **cayenne pepper**.
2. Simmer the beef in the **stock** with the **onion**, **red pepper** and **chilli** for 5 mins.
3. Add the **plantain** and enough water to cover the ingredients. Bring to the boil and simmer for 12 mins or until the beef is tender.
4. Stir through the **beans** and **kale**. Cook for a further 2 mins.
5. Season with salt, pepper and additional spice to taste.

3 5-a-day	2g SatFat	7g Fat	33g Protein	360 Cals

Weight | 520g

9g Fibre	42g Carbs

Chinese Sea Bass

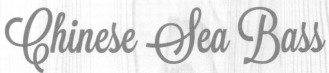

Dig out your steamer and whip up
this fresh fishy dish

Ingredients

120g	**Green Cabbage** (shredded)
140g	**Sea Bass** (raw fillet, sustainable)
½	**Green Chilli** (sliced)
1 inch	**Ginger** (grated)
1 clove	**Garlic** (sliced)
1 tbsp	**Sesame Oil**
2 tsp	**Soy Sauce**

Preparation

1. Steam the **cabbage** for 5 mins (in a steamer, or on the hob).

2. Place the **fish** on top of the cabbage, and sprinkle with the **chilli** and **ginger**. Steam until the fish is completely cooked (it will appear opaque).

3. In a separate pan, gently fry the **garlic** in 1 tbsp oil, stirring constantly until coloured.

4. Serve the cabbage topped with the fish, and drizzle with the fried garlic and **soy sauce**.

5. Delicious with basmati rice (optional, see page 178).

8g Carbs   **5g** Fibre

380 Cals   **31g** Protein   **25g** Fat   **5g** SatFat   **1** 5-a-day

Weight | 280g

Chunky Cottage Pie

Is anything more comforting than a hearty cottage pie? This one provides a third of your fibre needs too!

Ingredients

100g	**Beef Sirloin** (raw, lean, cubed)
2 tsp	**Olive Oil**
¼	**Onion** (diced)
1 clove	**Garlic** (minced)
½	**Carrot** (sliced)
40g	**Peas**
1 sprig	**Rosemary** (leaves, chopped)
1 sprig	**Thyme** (leaves, chopped)
100ml	**Beef Stock** (½ cube)
100g	**New Potatoes** (cubed)
60g	**Savoy Cabbage** (sliced)

Preparation

1. Fry the **beef** in 2 tsp **oil** for 5 mins with the **onion**, **garlic**, **carrot**, **peas** and **herbs**.

2. Pour in the **stock** and simmer for 15 mins, or until the beef is completely cooked.

3. Meanwhile, boil the **potatoes** for 10 mins or until soft, then lightly crush with a fork.

4. Boil or steam the **cabbage** for 4 mins, until tender. Serve the beef mixture topped with the potato, and the cabbage on the side.

| 2 5-a-day | 7g SatFat | 22g Fat | 29g Protein | 430 Cals | | 10g Fibre | 30g Carbs |

Weight | 440g

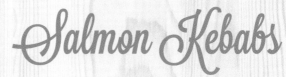

Salmon Kebabs

These healthy kebabs are perfect for the BBQ

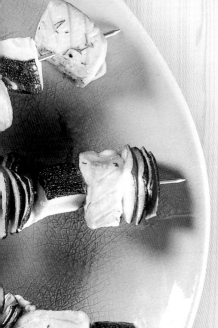

Ingredients

4 tsp	Olive Oil
½ tsp	Dijon Mustard
1	Lemon (juice only)
140g	Salmon (raw fillet, cubed)
⅓	Courgette (cubed)
⅓	Red Onion (cubed)
½	Yellow Pepper (cubed)
50g	Natural Yogurt
1 sprig	Dill (finely chopped)

Preparation

1. Mix 1 tbsp **oil**, **mustard**, salt & pepper and half the **lemon juice** in a bowl.

2. Coat the **salmon** with the mixture and allow to marinate in the fridge for 30 mins.

3. Fry the **courgette**, **onion** and **pepper** in 1 tsp oil for 4 mins until charred. Thread onto skewers with the salmon, to make kebabs.

4. Bake on a tray at 200°C for 8 mins, or until the salmon is completely cooked.

5. Meanwhile, mix the **yogurt**, remaining lemon juice, and **dill** in a bowl.

6. Serve the kebabs drizzled with the yogurt dressing.

13g Carbs

4g Fibre

490 Cals

36g Protein

33g Fat

6g SatFat

3 5-a-day

Weight | 320g

Beef Lo Mein

A nourishing noodle medley, propping up your protein intake by 40g

Ingredients

150g	**Beef Rump** (raw, lean, sliced)
2 tsp	**Soy Sauce**
2 tsp	**Chinese Rice Wine**
35g	dried **Rice Noodles**
1 tbsp	**Sesame Oil**
¼	**Red Pepper** (sliced)
40g	**Mangetout**
1	**Spring Onion** (sliced)
1	**Red Chilli** (sliced)
2 cloves	**Garlic** (sliced)
40g	**Beansprouts**
1 tbsp	**Oyster Sauce**

Preparation

1. Marinate the **beef** in 1 tsp **soy sauce** and 1 tsp **rice wine** for at least 30 mins.

2. Prepare the **rice noodles** according to the packet instructions, plunge into cold water, drain and set aside.

3. Fry the beef in ½ tbsp **oil** for 3 mins, or until well cooked. Remove from the pan.

4. Sauté the **pepper**, **mangetout**, **onion**, **chilli** and **garlic** in the remaining ½ tbsp oil, until the veg starts to soften.

5. Add the beef, **beansprouts**, noodles, 1 tsp rice wine, 1 tsp soy sauce and 1 tbsp **oyster sauce**. Serve & enjoy!

2 5-a-day	4g SatFat	19g Fat	40g Protein	505 Cals	4g Fibre	41g Carbs

Weight | 365g

Chicken & Cashew Stir-fry

One of our highest-protein dishes,
popping a whopping 64g!

Ingredients

2 tsp	**Olive Oil**
200g	**Chicken Breast** (raw, skinless, sliced)
½	**Red Chilli** (finely sliced)
1 inch	**Ginger** (finely chopped)
2	**Spring Onions** (sliced)
80g	**Mangetout**
2 tbsp	**Cashews**
160g	**Broccoli** (florets, blanched)
2 tsp	**Fish Sauce**
½	**Lemongrass** stalk (finely chopped)
½	**Lime** (juice only)
6	**Thai Basil** leaves (torn)
5	**Mint** leaves (chopped)

Preparation

1. Heat a wok until very hot. Add 2 tsp **oil** and the **chicken** strips.

2. After 2 mins, add the **chilli**, **ginger**, **spring onion**, **mangetout**, **cashews** and **broccoli**. Fry for 3 mins, or until the chicken is completely cooked.

3. Stir through the **fish sauce**, **lemongrass** and **lime juice**, and cook for a further minute.

4. Top with **Thai basil** and **mint** to serve.

16g Carbs

11g Fibre

505 Cals

64g Protein

21g Fat

4g SatFat

3 5-a-day

Weight | 340g

Fish Pie

A comforting dinner for those evenings when your taste buds need a bit of TLC!

Ingredients

120g	**Cauliflower** (small florets)
120g	**Butternut Squash** (cubed)
20g	**Parmesan** (grated)
¼	**Onion** (diced)
½	**Carrot** (finely chopped)
2 tsp	**Olive Oil**
1	handful **Spinach**
40g	**Tomato** (chopped)
1 sprig	**Dill** (chopped)
1 sprig	**Parsley** (large, chopped)
1 tbsp	**Whipping Cream**
140g	**Pollock** (raw fillet, cubed)
100g	**Prawns** (raw)
¼	**Lemon** (juice only)

Preparation

1. Steam the **cauliflower** and **squash** until tender. Mash with **parmesan**, salt & pepper.
2. Fry the **onion** and **carrot** in 2 tsp **oil** until soft. Stir in the **spinach** and allow to wilt.
3. Add the **tomato**, a splash of water and the **herbs**.
4. Cook until the tomato starts to break down, then fold in the **cream**.
5. Place the **fish** and **prawns** in a baking dish. Spoon the vegetable mixture evenly over the top.
6. Drizzle with **lemon juice** and top with the cauliflower mash. Bake at 180°C for 20 mins and serve.

5 5-a-day	9g SatFat	23g Fat	54g Protein	510 Cals		8g Fibre	24g Carbs

Weight | 500g

Mexican Chicken Mole

If you have a thing for chicken, you'll love this protein-packed one-pot wonder!

Ingredients

⅔	**Red Onion** (sliced)
½	**Red Pepper** (sliced)
1 tbsp	**Olive Oil**
2 cloves	**Garlic** (minced)
200g	**Chopped Tomatoes** (tinned)
80g	**Mixed Beans**
1 tbsp	**Mole Sauce**
200g	**Chicken Thighs** (raw, skinless, boneless)
1 sprig	**Parsley** (large, chopped)

Preparation

1. Gently fry the **onion** and **pepper** in 1 tbsp **oil** for 10 mins, until soft.
2. Add the **garlic** and cook for a further minute.
3. Stir in the **tomatoes**, **beans**, **mole sauce** and 150ml water, and bring to the boil.
4. Add the **chicken** and simmer for at least 30 mins, ensuring the chicken is thoroughly cooked.
5. Serve sprinkled with the chopped **parsley**.

31g Carbs

12g Fibre

515 Cals

52g Protein

20g Fat

4g SatFat

4 5-a-day

Weight | 450g

Chicken Jollof Rice

Ingredients

150g	**Chicken Thighs** (skinless, boneless, chopped)
2 tsp	**Rapeseed Oil**
pinch	**Cayenne Pepper**
¼	**Onion** (sliced)
½	**Green Chilli** (sliced)
1 clove	**Garlic** (minced)
1 inch	**Ginger** (grated)
300ml	**Chicken Stock** (½ cube)
80g	**Tomato** (chopped)
40g	**Green Beans** (halved)
20g	**Cabbage** (shredded)
1 tbsp	**Tomato Purée**
35g	uncooked **Brown Basmati Rice**
10g	**Dried Shrimp**
1 sprig	**Coriander** (chopped)
1 sprig	**Parsley** (chopped)

Preparation

1. In a frying pan, brown the **chicken** pieces in 1 tsp **oil** for a few mins, then set aside. To the same pan, add another 1 tsp oil, **cayenne pepper**, **onion**, **chilli**, **garlic** and **ginger**. Fry for 5 mins, or until the onions soften.

2. Boil the **stock**, add the onion mixture and reduce to a simmer.

3. In the frying pan, dry fry the **tomato**, **beans** and **cabbage** for 3 mins, then add to the stock. Stir the **tomato purée** through the uncooked **rice** until evenly coated, then add to the stock mixture together with the chicken and **shrimp**.

4. Cover and cook on a low heat for 20 mins, until the rice and chicken are cooked through. Serve topped with the **herbs**.

2½ 5-a-day	5g SatFat	25g Fat	40g Protein	540 Cals		7g Fibre	38g Carbs

Weight | 460g

Dijon Chicken with Mash

If you think mashed potato is marvellous, wait until you taste this parsnip & bean mash-up!

Ingredients

1	**Parsnip** (chunks)
80g	**Cannellini Beans**
200g	**Chicken Breast** (raw, skinless, diced)
2 tsp	**Olive Oil**
200ml	**Chicken Stock** (½ cube)
1 tsp	**Dijon Mustard**
50g	**Cream Cheese**
80g	**Broccoli** (florets)
80g	**Asparagus** (halved)
2 sprigs	**Tarragon** (chopped)

Preparation

1. Boil the **parsnip** (using water from cold). Simmer for 12 mins until soft, adding the **beans** for the final minute. Drain and mash.

2. Fry the **chicken** on a high heat in 2 tsp **oil** for 5 mins, or until golden. Transfer to a warm plate.

3. In the same pan, boil the **stock**, whisking in the **mustard** and **cheese**. Return the chicken to the pan and simmer for 10 mins, or until completely cooked.

4. Meanwhile, boil or steam the **veg** for 3 mins, until tender.

5. Serve sprinkled with **tarragon** and drizzled with sauce.

29g Carbs

14g Fibre

600 Cals

65g Protein

25g Fat

10g SatFat

4 5-a-day

Weight | 495g

Chicken, Kale & Chorizo

A delectable dish high in protein and packed full of iron

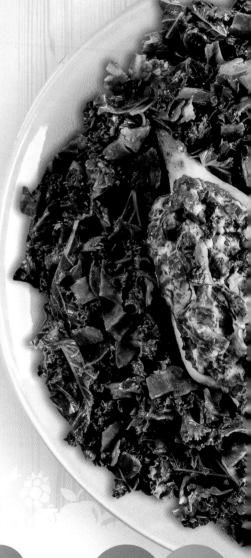

Ingredients

40g	**Roasted Red Pepper** (from jar, chopped)
50g	**Cream Cheese**
6	**Basil** leaves (torn)
150g	**Chicken Breast** (raw, skinless)
1 tbsp	**Olive Oil**
50g	**Chorizo** (small slices)
4	handfuls **Kale** (chopped)

Preparation

1. Mix the **pepper** with the **cheese** and **basil**. Cut a pocket into the **chicken breast** and spoon in the cheese mixture.

2. Rub 1 tbsp **oil** over the chicken and bake for 18 mins at 200°C, or until the chicken is thoroughly cooked.

3. Gently dry fry the **chorizo** until oils are released. Turn the heat up, add a good splash of water and the **kale.**

4. Cook until the kale has wilted, then serve topped with the chicken.

1½ 5-a-day	16g SatFat	43g Fat	54g Protein	630 Cals	5g Fibre	6g Carbs

Weight | 320g

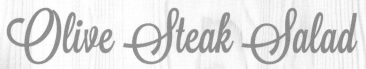

Olive Steak Salad

A perfect combination of steak, olives and sprouts

Ingredients

1 tsp	**Olive Oil**
100g	**Beef Sirloin** (raw, lean)
40g	**Alfalfa Sprouts**
1 sprig	**Dill** (finely chopped)
8	**Olives** (small, chopped)
80g	**Tomato** (chopped)
1	large handful **Watercress**
¼	**Lemon** (juice only)

Preparation

1. Heat the **oil** in a pan over a medium-high heat and fry the **steak** until well done on both sides, at least 4 mins. Remove pan from the heat.

2. Mix **all the salad ingredients** (except the lemon juice) and place on a plate.

3. Slice the steak into strips, and lay on top of the salad.

4. Drizzle with juices from the pan and the **lemon juice**.

3g Carbs

3g Fibre

225 Cals

26g Protein

12g Fat

3g SatFat

2 5-a-day

Weight | 285g

Mustard Chicken Salad

With 33g protein in one dish, this chicken and wholegrain mustard fusion is a great way to fill up

Ingredients

80g	**Chicken Breast**	(grilled, sliced)
2	handfuls **Mixed Salad Leaves**	
4	**Cherry Tomatoes**	(quartered)
80g	**Black Eye Beans**	(tinned)
1 sprig	**Tarragon**	(chopped)

Dressing

1 tsp	**Wholegrain Mustard**	
1 tsp	**White Wine Vinegar**	
2 tsp	**Olive Oil**	(extra virgin)

Preparation

1. Whisk the **dressing** together until mixed well.
2. Combine the **salad ingredients** and gently stir through the dressing.
3. Season with salt & pepper and serve.

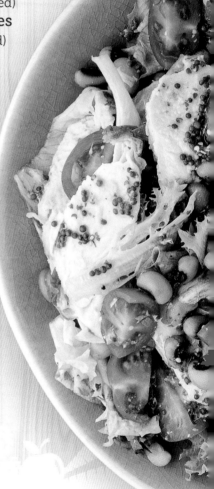

2 5-a-day	2g SatFat	11g Fat	33g Protein	305 Cals

Weight | 260g

5g Fibre	16g Carbs

Egg & Mackerel Salad

A creamy horseradish hit for the taste buds

Ingredients

2	handfuls **Mixed Salad Leaves**
40g	**Asparagus Tips** (blanched)
4	**Cherry Tomatoes** (halved)
1	**Egg** (hard boiled, sliced)
75g	**Smoked Mackerel**

Dressing

1 tbsp	**Greek Yogurt**
1 clove	**Garlic** (minced)
¼	**Lemon** (juice only)
1 tsp	**Horseradish Sauce**

Preparation

1. Layer the **salad leaves** and **asparagus** on a plate, then top with the **tomatoes**, **egg** and **mackerel**.

2. Whisk the **dressing** until well combined and drizzle over the salad.

3. Season with salt & pepper and serve.

5g Carbs

2g Fibre

370 Cals

28g Protein

26g Fat

6g SatFat

1½ 5-a-day

Weight | 295g

Tuna & Bean Salad

Packed with 44g protein and half of your 5-a-day

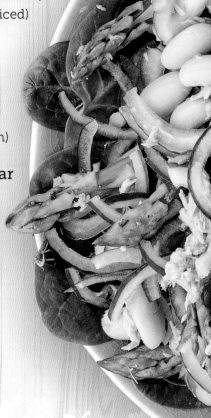

Ingredients

40g	**Asparagus Tips** (blanched)
80g	**Cannellini Beans** (tinned)
⅓	**Red Onion** (thinly sliced)
2	handfuls **Spinach**
140g	**Tuna** (tinned)

Dressing

1 sprig	**Dill** (chopped)
½ clove	**Garlic** (crushed)
1 tbsp	**Olive Oil** (extra virgin)
1 sprig	**Parsley** (large)
1 tbsp	**White Wine Vinegar**

Preparation

1. Mix **all the salad ingredients** and season with salt & pepper.
2. Whisk the **dressing** until well combined and gently stir through the salad.

2½ 5-a-day	2g SatFat	14g Fat	44g Protein	375 Cals

Weight | 345g

8g Fibre	17g Carbs

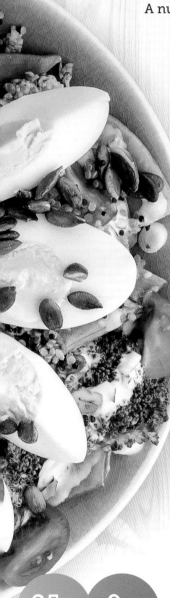

Egg & Quinoa Salad

A nutritious marriage of high-protein ingredients

Ingredients

40g	**Broccoli** (chopped)
4	**Cherry Tomatoes** (quartered)
80g	cooked **Quinoa**
1	**Spring Onion** (finely sliced)
40g	**Sugar Snap Peas** (halved)
1	**Egg** (hard boiled, quartered)
1 tbsp	**Pumpkin Seeds** (toasted)

Dressing

1 clove	**Garlic** (finely chopped)
¼	**Lemon** (juice only)
2 sprigs	**Parsley** (finely chopped)
1 tbsp	**Tahini**
1 tbsp	**Water**

Preparation

1. Boil or steam the **broccoli** for 3 mins, or until tender.
2. Mix **all the salad ingredients** except the egg and pumpkin seeds.
3. Whisk the **dressing** until well combined and stir through the salad.
4. Serve topped with the **egg** and scattered with **pumpkin seeds**.

25g Carbs

9g Fibre

390 Cals

24g Protein

22g Fat

4g SatFat

2 5-a-day

Weight | 370g

Thai Vegan Salad

No meat, no fish, no dairy... just 100% taste!

Ingredients

100g	**Tofu** (firm, cubed)
1 tsp	**Sesame Oil**
1/4	**Yellow Pepper** (matchsticks)
1/4	**Cucumber** (matchsticks)
1/3	**Courgette** (matchsticks)
2	**Spring Onions** (sliced)
40g	**Red Cabbage** (sliced)
2 sprigs	**Coriander** (chopped)
1	**Carrot** (matchsticks)
20g	**Radishes** (sliced)
40g	**Beansprouts**

Dressing

1 clove	**Garlic** (minced)
1/2 inch	**Ginger** (minced)
1/4	**Lime** (juice only)
2 tbsp	**Peanut Butter**
1 tbsp	**Rice Wine Vinegar**
1 tbsp	**Soy Sauce**

Preparation

1. Dry the **tofu** between paper towels. Rub with 1 tsp **oil** and bake for 45 mins at 180°C, until crispy.

2. Mix **all the other salad ingredients**.

3. Whisk the **dressing** and stir through the salad, topping with the tofu.

5 5-a-day   **4g** SatFat   **23g** Fat   **20g** Protein   **390** Cals   **10g** Fibre   **25g** Carbs

Weight | 560g

Warm Squash Salad

Smoky houmous is a great addition to this kale and squash salad

Ingredients

80g	**Butternut Squash** (cubed)
½	**Yellow Pepper** (sliced)
1 tbsp	**Olive Oil**
2	handfuls **Kale**
2 tbsp	**Pumpkin Seeds**

Dressing

80g	**Chickpeas** (tinned)
½ tsp	**Cumin** (ground)
1 clove	**Garlic** (minced)
¼	**Lemon** (juice only)
½ tsp	**Smoked Paprika**
1 tbsp	**Tahini**
2 tbsp	**Water**

Preparation

1. Bake the **squash** and **pepper** at 180°C with 1 tbsp **oil** for 20 mins.
2. Add the **kale** and cook for 5 mins more.
3. Meanwhile, blitz the **dressing** in a blender to make the houmous.
4. Serve the salad topped with the houmous & **pumpkin seeds**.

30g Carbs

13g Fibre

485 Cals

17g Protein

34g Fat

5g SatFat

3½ 5-a-day

Weight | 340g

Squash & Nut Salad

Go nuts for this wonderful mix

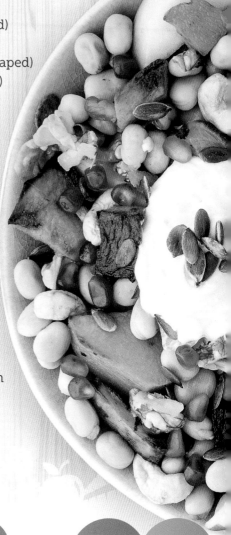

Ingredients

160g	**Butternut Squash**	(cubed)
1 tsp	**Olive Oil**	
1 tbsp	**Pomegranate Seeds**	(heaped)
40g	**Little Gem Lettuce**	(torn)
1 sprig	**Thyme**	(leaves, chopped)
80g	**Soya Beans**	(cooked)
1 tbsp	**Cashews**	(chopped)
1 tbsp	**Walnuts**	(chopped)
¼	**Red Apple**	(sliced)
1 tbsp	**Pumpkin Seeds**	

Dressing

1 clove	**Garlic**	
1 tsp	**Tahini**	
¼	**Lemon**	(juice only)
25g	**Greek Yogurt**	(fat free)

Preparation

1. Roast the **squash** in 1 tsp **oil** at 180°C for 25 mins.
2. When cooked, mix the squash with the **remaining salad ingredients**.
3. Whisk the **dressing** and spoon over the salad.

3½ 5-a-day · **4g** SatFat · **29g** Fat · **22g** Protein · **485** Cals

11g Fibre · **32g** Carbs

Weight | 385g

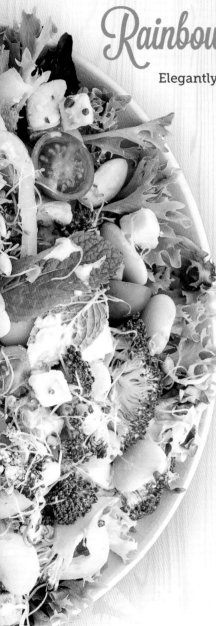

Rainbow Tahini Salad

Elegantly balanced with a tasty tahini dressing, this salad contains 6 of your 5-a-day!

Ingredients

1	**Spring Onion** (thinly sliced)
8	**Cherry Tomatoes** (halved)
1/2	**Yellow Pepper** (sliced)
80g	**Butter Beans** (tinned)
40g	**Broccoli** (chopped)
2 tbsp	**Sunflower Seeds**
5	**Mint** leaves (torn)
1	**Avocado** (cubed)
20g	**Alfalfa Sprouts**
2	handfuls **Salad Leaves**

Dressing

1 tbsp	**Tahini**
1/2	**Lemon** (juice only)

Preparation

1. Mix together **all the ingredients** except the salad leaves.
2. Arrange the **salad leaves** on a plate and top with the mixture.
3. Stir together the **dressing** and drizzle over the salad.

29g Carbs

21g Fibre

620 Cals

21g Protein

47g Fat

9g SatFat

6 5-a-day

Weight | 580g

Roots & Lentil Salad

A curious combination of roasted roots with a strawberry dressing

Ingredients

1	**Raw Beetroot** (peeled, cubed)
160g	**Butternut Squash** (peeled, cubed)
1	**Parsnip** (chopped)
1 clove	**Garlic** (minced)
1 tbsp	**Olive Oil**
2	handfuls **Watercress**
120g	cooked **Puy Lentils**
50g	**Goat's Cheese** (cubed)

Dressing

2 tsp	**Balsamic Vinegar**
½ tsp	**Dijon Mustard**
¼	**Lemon** (juice only)
2 tsp	**Olive Oil** (extra virgin)
1 tsp	**Red Wine Vinegar**
2	**Strawberries** (mashed)

Preparation

1. Roast the **beetroot**, **squash**, **parsnip** and **garlic** in 1 tbsp **oil** for 30 mins at 180°C.
2. Whisk the **dressing** well.
3. Add the **watercress** to the cooked veg, stir in the **lentils** and dressing, and serve topped with the **cheese**.

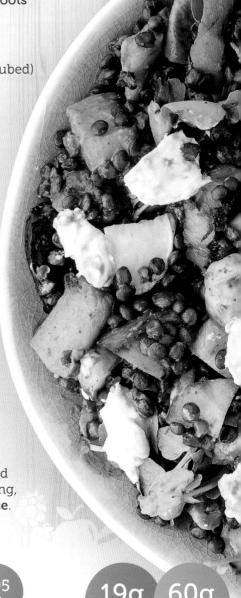

5 5-a-day	12g SatFat	37g Fat	29g Protein	695 Cals		19g Fibre	60g Carbs

Weight | 540g

Butternut Squash Soup

Slurp up 3 of your 5-a-day - the perfect light
lunch with plenty of nutrients

Ingredients

240g	**Butternut Squash** (peeled, cubed)
80g	**Chestnut Mushrooms** (halved)
½	**Onion** (chopped)
½	**Red Chilli** (sliced)
1 sprig	**Rosemary** (leaves, chopped)
1 sprig	**Thyme** (leaves, chopped)
400ml	**Vegetable Stock** (½ cube)

Preparation

1. Combine **all the ingredients** in a pan and bring to the boil.
2. Simmer for 20 mins, until the squash is cooked.
3. Whizz in a blender and serve.

28g Carbs

8g Fibre

140 Cals

5g Protein

1g Fat

0g SatFat

3 5-a-day

Weight | 480g

Veggie Stew

The easiest way to get all 5 of your 5-a-day!

Ingredients

80g	**Butternut Squash** (small cubes)
4	**Cherry Tomatoes** (halved)
300ml	**Vegetable Stock** (½ cube)
1 sprig	**Thyme** (leaves, chopped)
30g	dried **Red Split Lentils**
¼	**Yellow Pepper** (sliced)
80g	**Aubergine** (cubed)
½	**Celery** stalk (sliced)
½ tsp	**Smoked Paprika**
40g	**Leek** (thinly sliced)
1	**Carrot** (chopped)
1 clove	**Garlic** (minced)

Preparation

1. Add **all the ingredients** to a slow cooker and cook on medium for 3-4 hours.

5½ 5-a-day

0g SatFat

3g Fat

12g Protein

215 Cals

14g Fibre

38g Carbs

Weight | 480g

Parsnip Cauliflower Soup

Roasting cauliflower unlocks its hidden flavour!

Ingredients

160g	**Cauliflower** (florets)
2	**Parsnips** (cubed)
2 tsp	**Olive Oil**
¼	**Onion** (sliced)
2 cloves	**Garlic** (thinly sliced)
1 sprig	**Thyme** (leaves, chopped)
500ml	**Vegetable Stock** (½ cube)
30g	**Natural Yogurt**

Preparation

1. Coat the **cauliflower** and **parsnip** with 1 tsp **oil** and bake on a tray at 180°C for 20 mins.

2. Meanwhile, gently fry the **onion**, **garlic** and **thyme** in 1 tsp oil for 5 mins, until soft.

3. When the vegetables are cooked, pour the **stock** into the onion and garlic mixture, adding the roasted vegetables. Simmer for 5 mins.

4. Blend until smooth (adding extra water if the soup is too thick).

5. Serve topped with the **yogurt**.

33g Carbs

12g Fibre

270 Cals

9g Protein

12g Fat

2g SatFat

2½ 5-a-day

Weight | 500g

Beef & Pearl Barley Stew

A thick stew to warm your cockles
and delight your appetite

Ingredients

70g	**Stewing Beef** (raw, lean, cubed)
100g	**Chopped Tomatoes** (tinned)
1 sprig	**Rosemary** (leaves, chopped)
1 sprig	**Thyme** (leaves, chopped)
40g	**Mushrooms** (quartered)
1 tsp	**Worcestershire Sauce**
25g	uncooked **Pearl Barley**
½	**Celery** stalk (chopped)
300ml	**Beef Stock** (½ cube)
½	**Parsnip** (chopped)
1	**Carrot** (chopped)
¼	**Onion** (sliced)

Preparation

1. Add **all the ingredients** to a slow cooker.

2. Cook on medium for 4-6 hours, until the beef is soft and the pearl barley swollen.

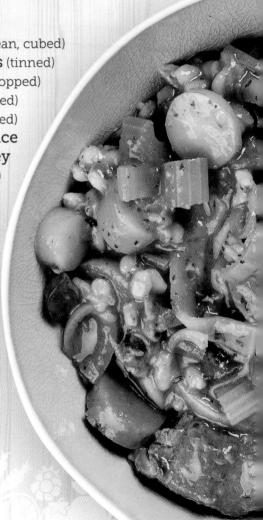

4 5-a-day	**1g** SatFat	**4g** Fat	**22g** Protein	**285** Cals

Weight | 485g

12g Fibre	**42g** Carbs

Chicken Tagine

Apricots add zesty sweetness to this lively dish

Ingredients

pinch	**Cinnamon** (ground)
pinch	**Coriander** (ground)
pinch	**Cumin** (ground)
75g	**Chicken Thighs** (raw, skinless, boneless)
40g	**Butternut Squash** (cubed)
1	**Carrot** (chopped)
400ml	**Chicken Stock** (½ cube)
80g	**Chickpeas** (tinned)
100g	**Chopped Tomatoes** (tinned)
3	**Dried Apricots** (chopped)
1 clove	**Garlic** (minced)
⅓	**Red Onion** (chopped)
1 sprig	**Parsley** (large, chopped)

Preparation

1. Rub the **spices** into the **chicken** and pan fry until brown on all sides.
2. Transfer to a slow cooker, adding **all the remaining ingredients** except the parsley.
3. Cook on low for 4 hours.
4. Serve topped with **parsley**.

37g Carbs

13g Fibre

295 Cals

25g Protein

6g Fat

1g SatFat

5½ 5-a-day

Weight | 505g

Jamaican Fish Stew

Ingredients

200g	**Haddock/Pollock** (raw fillet)
1/4	**Red Pepper** (sliced)
1/8	**Onion** (sliced)
1 clove	**Garlic** (minced)
1	**Spring Onion** (sliced)
pinch	**Paprika**
pinch	**Black Pepper** (ground)
pinch	**Thyme** (dried)
pinch	**Fish Seasoning**
1 tbsp	**Rapeseed Oil**
40g	**Tomato** (sliced)
1/2	**Green Chilli** (sliced)
1/2	**Carrot** (sliced)
1 tbsp	**Tomato Ketchup**

Preparation

1. Mix the **fish** with the **red pepper, onion, garlic** and **spring onion.**

2. Add the **paprika, black pepper, thyme** and **seasoning**. Marinate in the fridge for at least 30 mins (ideally overnight).

3. Remove the fish from the veg mixture. Brown in 1 tbsp **oil** for 2 mins on each side, then set aside.

4. Reduce the heat. Add the **tomato, chilli** and veg mix. Fry for 3 mins.

5. Stir in the **carrot, ketchup** and 200ml water. Boil for 6 mins, until the sauce reduces. Add the fish, cover, and simmer for 2 mins (or until the fish is thoroughly cooked). Serve & enjoy!

2 5-a-day	1g SatFat	13g Fat	38g Protein	325 Cals		5g Fibre	14g Carbs

Weight | 330g

African Bean Stew

Get half your 5-a-day, and a third of your fibre needs with this beany beauty!

Ingredients

¼	**Onion** (diced)
1 tbsp	**Rapeseed Oil**
120g	**Tomatoes** (chopped)
2 tsp	**Ground Crayfish**
160g	**Black Eye Beans**
pinch	**Cayenne Pepper**
200ml	**Vegetable Stock** (½ cube)

Preparation

1. Fry the **onion** in 1 tbsp **oil** for 8 mins, or until slightly browned.

2. Add the **tomato** and **ground crayfish**. Keep stirring for 5 mins, until thickened.

3. Mix through the **beans**, **cayenne pepper** and **stock**. Bring to the boil.

4. Reduce heat and simmer for 10 mins, then serve.

35g Carbs

10g Fibre

335 Cals

14g Protein

14g Fat

1g SatFat

2½ 5-a-day

Weight | 350g

Carrot & Lentil Soup

Chilli & spices give this carrot soup a gentle kick

Ingredients

1 tsp	**Cumin Seeds**
1 tbsp	**Olive Oil**
1½	**Carrots** (chopped)
1	**Celery** stalk (chopped)
¼	**Onion** (chopped)
1 clove	**Garlic** (minced)
½	**Red Chilli** (sliced)
30g	dried **Red Split Lentils**
400ml	**Vegetable Stock** (½ cube)
50g	**Greek Yogurt**
1 sprig	**Coriander** (chopped)

Preparation

1. Dry fry the **cumin seeds** in a saucepan until aromatic.

2. Add 1 tbsp **oil**, the **vegetables**, **garlic**, **chilli** and **lentils**, and fry for 3 mins.

3. Pour in the **stock**, bring to the boil and simmer for 15 mins, or until the lentils are swollen.

4. Blend until smooth if desired, or leave as a lovely broth.

5. Stir through the **yogurt** and serve topped with **coriander**.

3 5-a-day	4g SatFat	18g Fat	12g Protein	335 Cals	9g Fibre	34g Carbs

Weight | 475g

Tuscan Tomato Soup

This hearty, wholesome soup contains all 5 of your 5-a-day
and over half of your daily fibre needs!

Ingredients

40g	**Leeks** (thinly sliced)
½	**Celery** stalk (chopped)
1	**Carrot** (chopped)
1 clove	**Garlic** (minced)
1 sprig	**Rosemary** (leaves, chopped)
pinch	**Paprika**
1 tbsp	**Olive Oil**
200g	**Chopped Tomatoes** (tinned)
500ml	**Vegetable Stock** (½ cube)
80g	**Butter Beans** (tinned)
80g	**Cannellini Beans** (tinned)
1	handful **Kale**

Preparation

1. Fry the **leek, celery, carrot, garlic, rosemary** and **paprika** in 1 tbsp **oil** for 10 mins, until the veg softens.

2. Pour in the **tomatoes** and **stock**. Bring to the boil, then simmer for 10 mins.

3. Add the **beans** and bring back to the boil.

4. Finally, add the **kale**, cook for 1 min, then serve.

39g Carbs

17g Fibre

340 Cals

15g Protein

15g Fat

2g SatFat

5 5-a-day

Weight | 660g

Sausage Bean Broth

Simmering herbs create a flavoursome broth,
worthy of a tasty sausage

Ingredients

1	Pork Sausage
1/4	Onion (diced)
1 clove	Garlic (finely sliced)
1 sprig	Rosemary (leaves, chopped)
1/2	Celery stalk (finely sliced)
80g	Cabbage (shredded)
1/2	Carrot (diced)
1 tsp	Olive Oil
300ml	Chicken Stock (1/2 cube)
1 sprig	Thyme (leaves, chopped)
1	Bay Leaf
80g	Butter Beans (tinned)

Preparation

1. Dry fry or grill the **sausage** for 7 mins, until the edges brown. Slice and set aside.

2. Sauté the **onion**, **garlic**, **rosemary**, **celery**, **cabbage** and **carrot** in 1 tsp **oil** for 5 mins.

3. Pour in the **stock** with the **thyme**, **bay leaf** and sausage. Simmer gently for 20 mins, or until the sausage is thoroughly cooked.

4. Stir in the **beans**, heat through and serve.

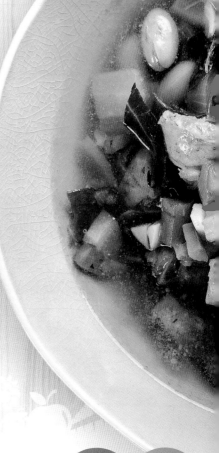

3½ 5-a-day	7g SatFat	23g Fat	16g Protein	375 Cals

14g Fibre	28g Carbs

Weight | 465g

Spring Chicken Soup

This tasty chicken soup packs a whopping 56g protein and 3 of your 5-a-day!

Ingredients

1 clove	**Garlic** (minced)
1/6	**Red Onion** (sliced)
1/2	**Carrot** (sliced)
1/2	**Celery** stalk (sliced)
2 tsp	**Olive Oil**
400ml	**Chicken Stock** (1/2 cube)
200g	**Chicken Breast** (raw, skinless, sliced)
80g	**Broccoli** (small florets)
20g	**Cabbage** (sliced)
40g	**Peas**
1 sprig	**Parsley** (large, chopped)
1 sprig	**Thyme** (leaves, chopped)

Preparation

1. Fry the **garlic**, **onion**, **carrot** and **celery** in 2 tsp **oil**, until softened.
2. Pour in the **stock** and **chicken**. Simmer for 8 mins, or until the chicken is cooked through.
3. Stir in the **broccoli** and cook for 2 mins before folding in the **cabbage**, **peas** and **herbs**.
4. Heat for a final 2 min before serving.

14g Carbs

9g Fibre

385 Cals

56g Protein

12g Fat

2g SatFat

3 5-a-day

Weight | 595g

Fragrant Crab Soup

This balanced blend of flavours has the unmistakable taste of Thailand

Ingredients

1 clove	Garlic	(minced)
1	Spring Onion	(sliced)
½ inch	Ginger	(grated)
1 tsp	Chilli Oil	
¼	Red Pepper	(thinly sliced)
300ml	Vegetable Stock	(½ cube)
150ml	Coconut Milk	(tinned)
2	Kaffir Lime Leaves	(torn)
¼	Lime	(juice & zest)
100g	Crab	(tinned)
1 sprig	Coriander	(chopped)
20g	Cabbage	(shredded)
40g	Pak Choi	(chopped)

Preparation

1. Fry the **garlic, spring onion** and **ginger** in 1 tsp **chilli oil** for 3 mins.
2. Add the **pepper** for 3 more mins.
3. Pour in the **stock** and **coconut milk**, and bring to the boil.
4. Stir in the **kaffir lime leaves, lime juice & zest**. Simmer for 5 mins.
5. Mix through the **crab, coriander, cabbage** and **pak choi**.
6. Simmer for 7 mins, then serve.

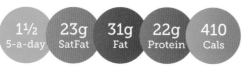

| 1½ 5-a-day | 23g SatFat | 31g Fat | 22g Protein | 410 Cals | | 4g Fibre | 12g Carbs |

Weight | 480g

Nigerian Chicken Stew

Ingredients

120g	Tomato
1/4	Habanero Chilli
1/2	Onion
2	Chicken Drumsticks (raw)
400ml	Chicken Stock (1/2 cube)
pinch	Thyme (dried)
pinch	Curry Powder
1 tbsp	Rapeseed Oil
1 tbsp	Tomato Purée

Preparation

1. Blend the **tomato**, **chilli** and **onion** in a food processor, then heat in a pan to thicken.

2. In a separate pan, cover the **chicken drumsticks** with the **stock**. Stir in the **thyme** and **curry powder**. Boil for 15 mins, or until cooked, then reserve the cooking liquid.

3. Brush the cooked chicken with 1 tsp **oil** and bake at 200°C for 15 mins, until crisp.

4. Once the tomato mixture is thickened, add the **tomato purée**. Transfer to a frying pan and fry in the remaining 2 tsp oil for 8 mins, stirring constantly.

5. Add 200ml cooking liquid, bubble on a high heat for 3 mins to reduce the liquid. Spoon the stew over the chicken and serve.

13g Carbs

4g Fibre

505 Cals

40g Protein

33g Fat

7g SatFat

2 5-a-day

Weight | 400g

Groundnut Soup

This rich bowl of chicken yumminess provides a peanutty protein punch of a staggering 58g!

Ingredients

½ tsp	**Chilli Powder**
pinch	**Thyme** (dried)
1 inch	**Ginger** (grated)
1 clove	**Garlic** (minced)
1 tbsp	**Groundnut or Olive Oil**
200g	**Chicken Breast** (raw, skinless, diced)
¼	**Onion** (diced)
¼	**Red Pepper** (chopped)
300ml	**Chicken Stock** (½ cube)
2 tbsp	**Peanut Butter**
40g	**Tomato** (chopped)
1	handful **Baby Spinach**

Preparation

1. Use the **chilli powder**, **thyme**, **ginger**, **garlic**, 1 tbsp **oil**, salt and pepper to coat the **chicken**.

2. Allow to marinate for at least 15 mins.

3. Fry the chicken mixture until the chicken starts to brown.

4. Add the **onion** and **pepper** for a further 5 mins. Then pour in the **stock**, **peanut butter** and **tomato**.

5. Bring to the boil, cover and simmer for 15 mins. Remove the lid and simmer uncovered for 5 mins more, or until the chicken is completely cooked.

6. Stir in the **spinach** and serve.

2	5g	30g	58g	550
5-a-day	SatFat	Fat	Protein	Cals

Weight | 420g

5g	12g
Fibre	Carbs

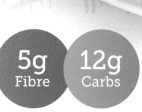

Lamb & Rosemary Stew

After several hours in the slow cooker, the lamb
will be ready to melt in your mouth!

Ingredients

1 tsp	Plain Flour
100g	Stewing Lamb (raw, lean, diced)
1 tbsp	Olive Oil
1 tsp	Tomato Purée
50ml	Red Wine
250ml	Beef Stock (½ cube)
½	Carrot (chopped)
½	Celery stalk (chopped)
1 clove	Garlic (minced)
¼	Onion (thinly sliced)
25g	uncooked Pearl Barley
1 sprig	Rosemary (leaves, chopped)
80g	Broccoli (small florets)
20g	Cabbage (sliced)

Preparation

1. Season the **flour** with salt & pepper,
   then use it to coat the **lamb**.

2. Fry the lamb in 1 tbsp **oil** until browned.
   Transfer to a slow cooker.

3. In the same pan, mix the **tomato purée**,
   wine and **stock**. Bring to the boil.

4. Pour the mixture into the slow cooker. Add the
   remaining ingredients except cabbage and
   broccoli. Cook on low for 4-6 hours.

5. When the stew is ready, boil or steam
   the **broccoli** and **cabbage** for 3 mins.
   Stir through and serve.

37g Carbs | **12g** Fibre

575 Cals | **35g** Protein | **28g** Fat | **9g** SatFat | **3** 5-a-day

Weight | 445g

Palm Nut Soup

Slurp up this lovely beefy bowlful!

Ingredients

100g	**Beef Sirloin** (raw, lean, chunks)
400ml	**Chicken Stock** (½ cube)
¼	**Onion** (sliced)
1 clove	**Garlic** (sliced)
pinch	**Smoked Paprika**
½ tsp	**Black Pepper** (ground)
75g	**Palm Fruit Concentrate**
80g	**Tomato** (chopped)
10g	**Dried Shrimp**
2	handfuls **Spinach**

Preparation

1. Boil the **meat** in the **stock** for 5 mins, along with the **onion, garlic, paprika** and **black pepper**.

2. Add the **palm fruit, tomato** and **dried shrimp**. Simmer for 10 mins.

3. Stir through the **spinach**, heat gently for a further 5 mins (or until the beef is thoroughly cooked) and serve.

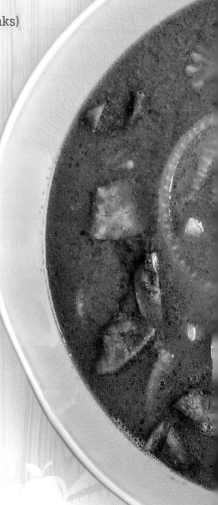

2	6g	45g	33g	590
5-a-day	SatFat	Fat	Protein	Cals

Weight | 580g

5g	14g
Fibre	Carbs

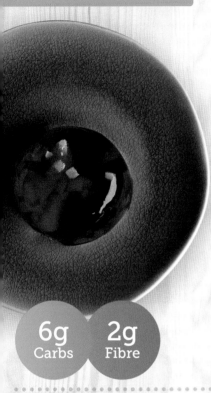

Berries & Jelly

Ingredients

1 sachet **Jelly Powder** (sugar free)
40g   **Strawberries** (diced)
40g   **Blueberries**

Preparation

1. Prepare the **Jelly liquid** according to packet instructions.
2. Lay the **fruit** in a small, individual mould, pour in 70ml jelly liquid and place in the fridge to set.
3. Serve and enjoy!

6g Carbs   **2g** Fibre

| 35 Cals | 2g Protein | 0g Fat | 0g SatFat | 1 5-a-day |

Weight | 150g

Kale Crisps

Ingredients

2   handfuls **Kale**
pinch   **Smoked Paprika**
¼   **Lemon** (juice & zest)

Preparation

1. Mix the **kale** with 1 tsp **oil**, **paprika** and salt & pepper.
2. Spread out on a baking tray and bake at 150°C for 15 mins.
3. Sprinkle with **lemon juice & zest**.

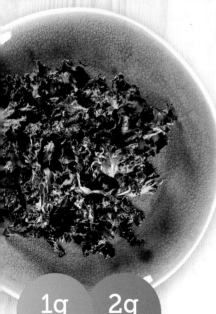

1g Carbs   **2g** Fibre

| 55 Cals | 2g Protein | 5g Fat | 1g SatFat | ½ 5-a-day |

Weight | 30g

Rosemary Olives

Ingredients

1 clove	**Garlic**	(finely chopped)
¼	**Lemon**	(juice & zest)
50g	**Olives**	(tinned in brine)
1 sprig	**Rosemary**	(leaves, chopped)

Preparation

1. Jumble **everything** together and serve.

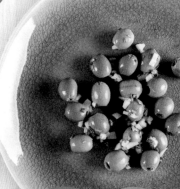

1 5-a-day	1g SatFat	6g Fat	1g Protein	60 Cals

2g Fibre	1g Carbs

Weight | 70g

Vanilla Berries

Ingredients

40g	**Blueberries**
40g	**Raspberries**
40g	**Strawberries** (quartered)
1 tsp	**Icing Sugar**
1 tbsp	**Orange Juice**
⅓	**Vanilla Pod** (seeds)

Preparation

1. Place the **fruit** in a bowl and stir through the **remaining ingredients**.
2. Leave to stand for 5 mins before serving.

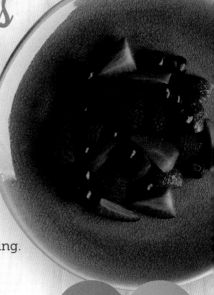

1½ 5-a-day	0g SatFat	1g Fat	1g Protein	60 Cals

4g Fibre	13g Carbs

Weight | 135g

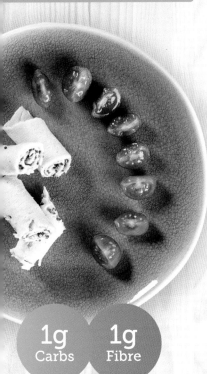

Turkey Rolls

Ingredients

1 tsp	**Wholegrain Mustard**
45g	cooked **Turkey** (thinly sliced)
2	**Cherry Tomatoes** (quartered)

Preparation

1. Spread **mustard** on one side of the **turkey**.
2. Roll into a sausage shape, with the mustard on the inside.
3. Cut in half and serve with the **tomatoes**.

65 Cals	11g Protein	1g Fat	0g SatFat	0 5-a-day

Weight | 70g

1g Carbs   1g Fibre

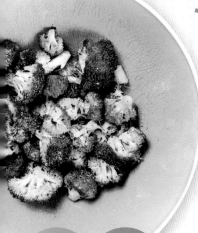

Spiced Broccoli

Ingredients

80g	**Broccoli** (florets, chopped)
pinch	**Chilli Flakes**
1 clove	**Garlic** (finely sliced)
1/4	**Lemon** (juice only)

Preparation

1. Fry the **broccoli**, **chilli flakes** and **garlic** in 1 tsp **oil** for 5 mins.
2. Serve drizzled with **lemon juice**.

65 Cals	4g Protein	4g Fat	1g SatFat	1 5-a-day

Weight | 90g

3g Carbs   3g Fibre

Pineapple Crispbread

Ingredients

1 slice	Rye Crispbread
30g	Cottage Cheese
20g	Pineapple

Preparation

1. Spread the **crispbread** with **cottage cheese** and top with the **pineapple**.

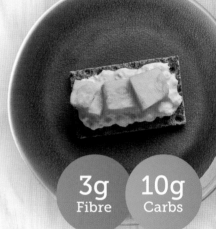

0 5-a-day	1g SatFat	2g Fat	4g Protein	70 Cals	3g Fibre	10g Carbs

Weight | 60g

Celery & Nut Butter

Ingredients

1	Celery stalk
2 tsp	Almond Butter

Preparation

1. Half the **celery** stalk and serve filled with the **almond butter**.

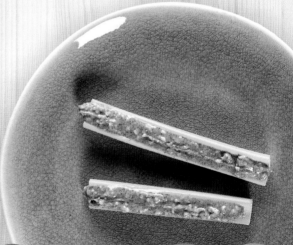

1 5-a-day	0g SatFat	6g Fat	3g Protein	70 Cals	2g Fibre	1g Carbs

Weight | 90g

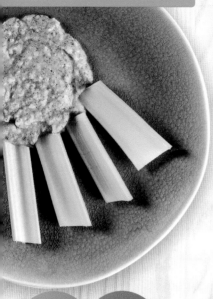

Butterbean Dip

Ingredients

80g	**Butter Beans** (tinned)
pinch	**Cumin** (ground)
1 clove	**Garlic**
¼	**Lemon** (juice only)
5	**Mint** leaves
1	**Celery** stalk (quartered)

Preparation

1. Whizz **all ingredients** (except celery) in a blender. If too thick, add water.
2. Serve with the **celery**.

12g Carbs **6g** Fibre

75 Cals **6g** Protein **1g** Fat **0g** SatFat **2** 5-a-day

Weight | 180g

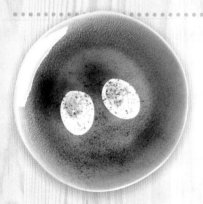

Devilled Eggs

Ingredients

1	**Egg** (hard boiled, peeled)
1 tsp	**Mayonnaise**
¼ tsp	**Dijon Mustard**
dash	**Tabasco**
pinch	**Paprika**

Preparation

1. Cut the **egg** in half, scoop out the yolk and keep the white to one side.
2. Mash the yolk with the **mayonnaise**, **mustard** and **Tabasco**.
3. Spoon the mixture into the egg white and sprinkle with **paprika**.

1g Carbs **0g** Fibre

95 Cals **8g** Protein **7g** Fat **2g** SatFat **0** 5-a-day

Weight | 65g

Soya Beans

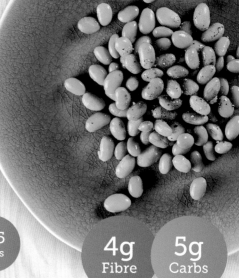

Ingredients

80g **Soya Beans**

Preparation

1. Boil the **soya beans** in salted water for 2 mins.
2. Serve sprinkled with salt & pepper.

1 5-a-day	1g SatFat	6g Fat	8g Protein	115 Cals

4g Fibre   **5g** Carbs

Weight | 80g

Roasted Pumpkin Seeds

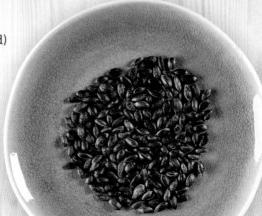

Ingredients

pinch **Cinnamon** (ground)
pinch **Nutmeg**
2 tbsp **Pumpkin Seeds**

Preparation

1. Combine **all the ingredients** and bake at 150°C for 15 mins, stirring half way.

0 5-a-day	2g SatFat	9g Fat	5g Protein	120 Cals

2g Fibre   **4g** Carbs

Weight | 15g

Avofennel Smoothie

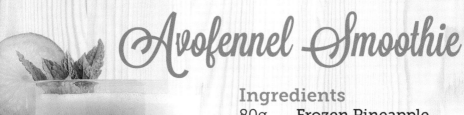

Ingredients

80g	**Frozen Pineapple**
1/4	**Avocado** (no skin)
40g	**Fennel**
1/2 tsp	**Chia Seeds**
1/2	**Lime** (juice only)
240ml	Water

11g Carbs **5g** Fibre

125 Cals **2g** Protein **8g** Fat **1g** SatFat **2** 5-a-day

Weight | 415g

Pick up a Pepper Smoothie

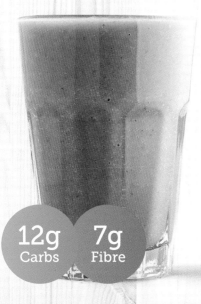

Ingredients

1/2	**Pear** (cored)
1/4	**Avocado** (no skin)
1/2	**Celery** stalk
2	handfuls **Spinach**
1/4	**Yellow Pepper** (small)
1/4	**Lime** (juice only)
140ml	Water
3	Ice Cubes

12g Carbs **7g** Fibre

125 Cals **3g** Protein **7g** Fat **1g** SatFat **3** 5-a-day

Weight | 425g

Tuna Lettuce Wraps

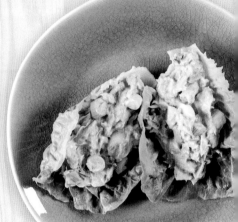

Ingredients

70g   **Tuna** (tinned)
1   **Spring Onion** (sliced)
2 tsp **Mayonnaise**
2   **Little Gem Lettuce** leaves

Preparation

1. Stir together the **tuna**, **onion** and **mayonnaise**.

2. Spoon the mixture into the **lettuce** leaves and serve.

½ 5-a-day   **1g** SatFat   **6g** Fat   **18g** Protein   **135** Cals   **1g** Fibre   **2g** Carbs

Weight | 125g

Cheesy Oatcakes

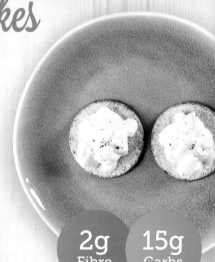

Ingredients

⅛   **Cucumber** (chopped)
50g **Cottage Cheese**
2   **Oatcakes**

Preparation

1. Combine the **cucumber** with the **cheese**, and serve on the **oatcakes**.

½ 5-a-day   **3g** SatFat   **7g** Fat   **7g** Protein   **150** Cals   **2g** Fibre   **15g** Carbs

Weight | 110g

Mozzarella & Tomato

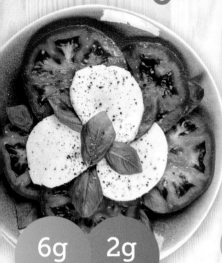

Ingredients

200g **Beef Tomato** (sliced across the core)

50g **Mozzarella** (thickly sliced)

10 **Basil** leaves

Preparation

1. Layer the **tomato, mozzarella** and **basil** on a plate and serve.

| 6g Carbs | 2g Fibre | | 155 Cals | 10g Protein | 10g Fat | 7g SatFat | 1 5-a-day |

Weight | 250g

Guacamole

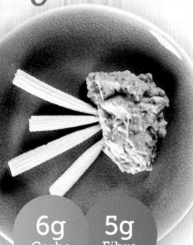

Ingredients

½ Avocado

pinch Chilli Flakes

1 sprig Coriander

¼ Lime (juice only)

⅙ Red Onion

40g Tomato (deseeded)

40g Baby Corn

Preparation

1. Blitz **all the ingredients** except the baby corn in a food processor.

2. Serve with the **baby corn.**

| 6g Carbs | 5g Fibre | | 165 Cals | 3g Protein | 14g Fat | 3g SatFat | 2 5-a-day |

Weight | 185g

Spicy Chickpeas

Ingredients

80g	**Chickpeas** (tinned)	
pinch	**Cumin** (ground)	
pinch	**Smoked Paprika**	
2 tsp	**Olive Oil**	

Preparation

1. Combine the **chickpeas** with the **spices**, 2 tsp **oil** and salt & pepper.
2. Bake at 180°C for 25 mins, or until the chickpeas are crispy.

| 1 5-a-day | 1g SatFat | 11g Fat | 6g Protein | 170 Cals | | 5g Fibre | 14g Carbs |

Weight | 50g

Maple Yogurt & Almonds

Ingredients

2 tbsp	**Almonds**
50g	**Natural Yogurt**
1 tsp	**Maple Syrup**

Preparation

1. Toast the **almonds** in a dry frying pan over a medium heat, until aromatic.
2. Fold the toasted almonds into the **yogurt** and serve drizzled with the **maple syrup**.

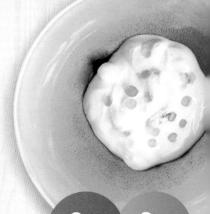

| 0 5-a-day | 2g SatFat | 13g Fat | 6g Protein | 170 Cals | | 2g Fibre | 8g Carbs |

Weight | 75g

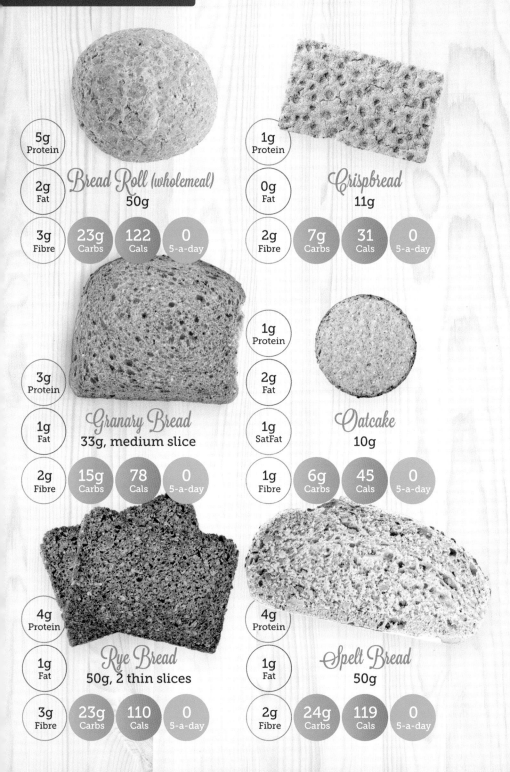

Bread Roll (wholemeal)
50g

- 5g Protein
- 2g Fat
- 3g Fibre
- 23g Carbs
- 122 Cals
- 0 5-a-day

Crispbread
11g

- 1g Protein
- 0g Fat
- 2g Fibre
- 7g Carbs
- 31 Cals
- 0 5-a-day

Granary Bread
33g, medium slice

- 3g Protein
- 1g Fat
- 2g Fibre
- 15g Carbs
- 78 Cals
- 0 5-a-day

Oatcake
10g

- 1g Protein
- 2g Fat
- 1g SatFat
- 1g Fibre
- 6g Carbs
- 45 Cals
- 0 5-a-day

Rye Bread
50g, 2 thin slices

- 4g Protein
- 1g Fat
- 3g Fibre
- 23g Carbs
- 110 Cals
- 0 5-a-day

Spelt Bread
50g

- 4g Protein
- 1g Fat
- 2g Fibre
- 24g Carbs
- 119 Cals
- 0 5-a-day

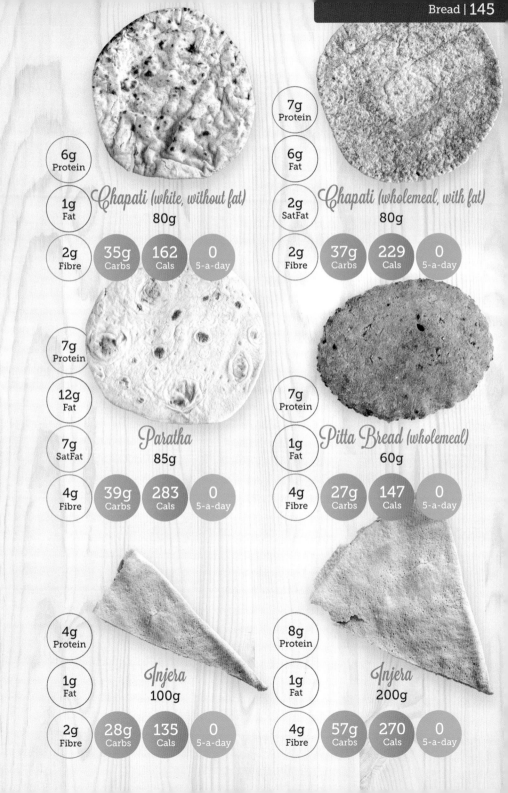

Chapati (white, without fat)
80g

6g Protein
1g Fat
2g Fibre
35g Carbs
162 Cals
0 5-a-day

Chapati (wholemeal, with fat)
80g

7g Protein
6g Fat
2g SatFat
2g Fibre
37g Carbs
229 Cals
0 5-a-day

Paratha
85g

7g Protein
12g Fat
7g SatFat
4g Fibre
39g Carbs
283 Cals
0 5-a-day

Pitta Bread (wholemeal)
60g

7g Protein
1g Fat
4g Fibre
27g Carbs
147 Cals
0 5-a-day

Injera
100g

4g Protein
1g Fat
2g Fibre
28g Carbs
135 Cals
0 5-a-day

Injera
200g

8g Protein
1g Fat
4g Fibre
57g Carbs
270 Cals
0 5-a-day

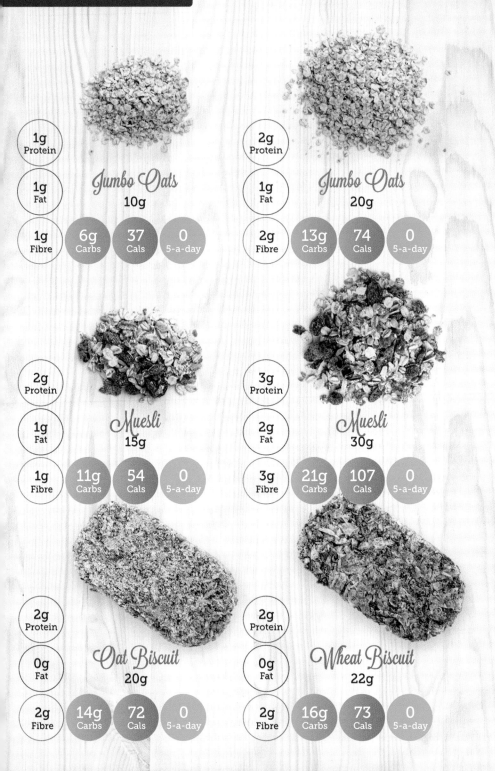

Jumbo Oats
10g

1g Protein
1g Fat
1g Fibre
6g Carbs
37 Cals
0 5-a-day

Jumbo Oats
20g

2g Protein
1g Fat
2g Fibre
13g Carbs
74 Cals
0 5-a-day

Muesli
15g

2g Protein
1g Fat
1g Fibre
11g Carbs
54 Cals
0 5-a-day

Muesli
30g

3g Protein
2g Fat
3g Fibre
21g Carbs
107 Cals
0 5-a-day

Oat Biscuit
20g

2g Protein
0g Fat
2g Fibre
14g Carbs
72 Cals
0 5-a-day

Wheat Biscuit
22g

2g Protein
0g Fat
2g Fibre
16g Carbs
73 Cals
0 5-a-day

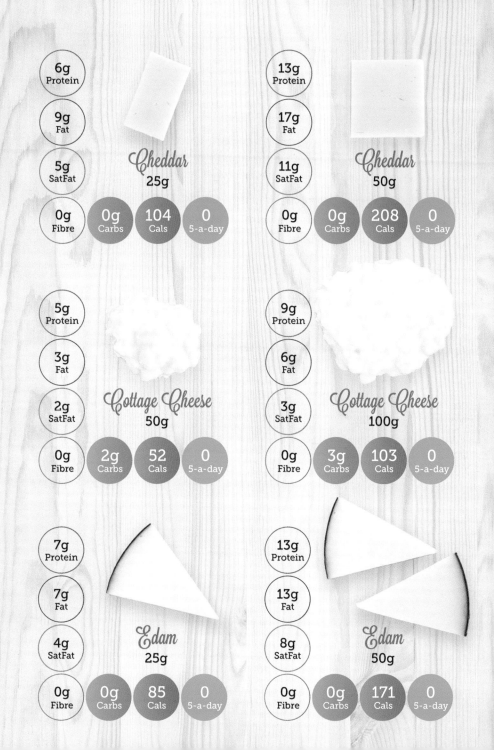

6g Protein

9g Fat

5g SatFat

0g Fibre

Cheddar
25g

0g Carbs

104 Cals

0 5-a-day

13g Protein

17g Fat

11g SatFat

0g Fibre

Cheddar
50g

0g Carbs

208 Cals

0 5-a-day

5g Protein

3g Fat

2g SatFat

0g Fibre

Cottage Cheese
50g

2g Carbs

52 Cals

0 5-a-day

9g Protein

6g Fat

3g SatFat

0g Fibre

Cottage Cheese
100g

3g Carbs

103 Cals

0 5-a-day

7g Protein

7g Fat

4g SatFat

0g Fibre

Edam
25g

0g Carbs

85 Cals

0 5-a-day

13g Protein

13g Fat

8g SatFat

0g Fibre

Edam
50g

0g Carbs

171 Cals

0 5-a-day

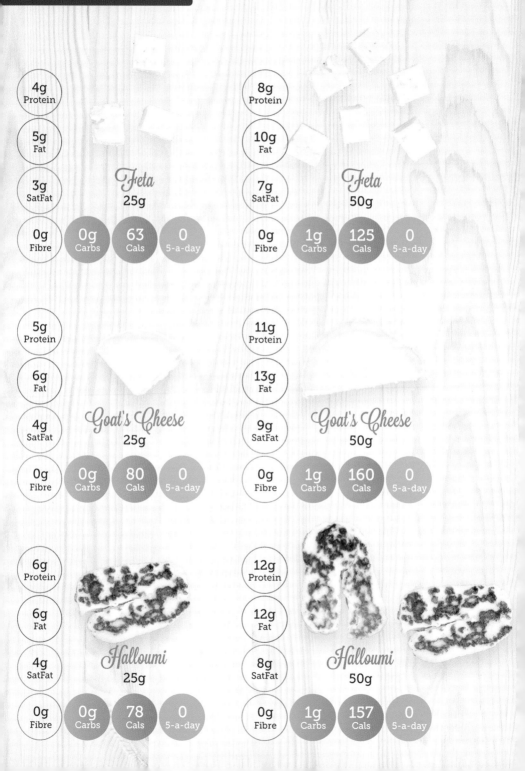

4g Protein

5g Fat

3g SatFat

0g Fibre

Feta
25g

0g Carbs

63 Cals

0 5-a-day

8g Protein

10g Fat

7g SatFat

0g Fibre

Feta
50g

1g Carbs

125 Cals

0 5-a-day

5g Protein

6g Fat

4g SatFat

0g Fibre

Goat's Cheese
25g

0g Carbs

80 Cals

0 5-a-day

11g Protein

13g Fat

9g SatFat

0g Fibre

Goat's Cheese
50g

1g Carbs

160 Cals

0 5-a-day

6g Protein

6g Fat

4g SatFat

0g Fibre

Halloumi
25g

0g Carbs

78 Cals

0 5-a-day

12g Protein

12g Fat

8g SatFat

0g Fibre

Halloumi
50g

1g Carbs

157 Cals

0 5-a-day

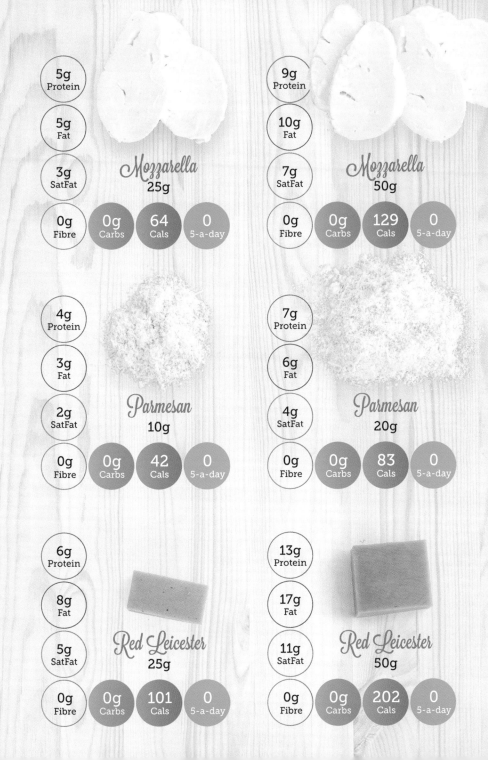

Mozzarella
25g

5g Protein
5g Fat
3g SatFat
0g Fibre
0g Carbs
64 Cals
0 5-a-day

Mozzarella
50g

9g Protein
10g Fat
7g SatFat
0g Fibre
0g Carbs
129 Cals
0 5-a-day

Parmesan
10g

4g Protein
3g Fat
2g SatFat
0g Fibre
0g Carbs
42 Cals
0 5-a-day

Parmesan
20g

7g Protein
6g Fat
4g SatFat
0g Fibre
0g Carbs
83 Cals
0 5-a-day

Red Leicester
25g

6g Protein
8g Fat
5g SatFat
0g Fibre
0g Carbs
101 Cals
0 5-a-day

Red Leicester
50g

13g Protein
17g Fat
11g SatFat
0g Fibre
0g Carbs
202 Cals
0 5-a-day

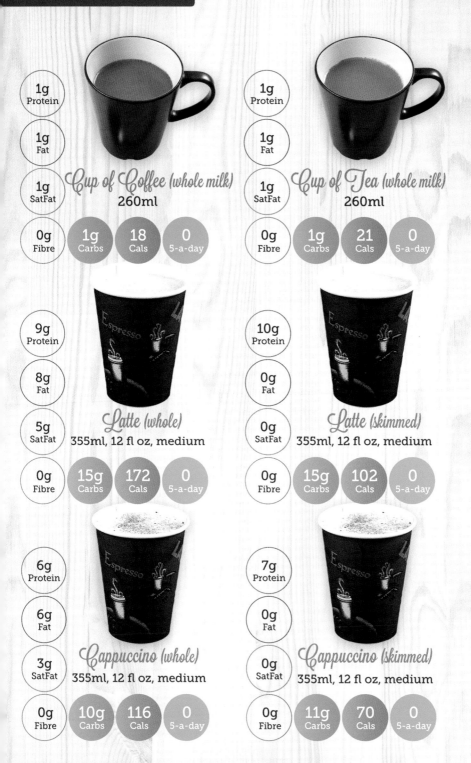

Cup of Coffee *(whole milk)*
260ml

1g Protein
1g Fat
1g SatFat
0g Fibre
1g Carbs
18 Cals
0 5-a-day

Cup of Tea *(whole milk)*
260ml

1g Protein
1g Fat
1g SatFat
0g Fibre
1g Carbs
21 Cals
0 5-a-day

Latte *(whole)*
355ml, 12 fl oz, medium

9g Protein
8g Fat
5g SatFat
0g Fibre
15g Carbs
172 Cals
0 5-a-day

Latte *(skimmed)*
355ml, 12 fl oz, medium

10g Protein
0g Fat
0g SatFat
0g Fibre
15g Carbs
102 Cals
0 5-a-day

Cappuccino *(whole)*
355ml, 12 fl oz, medium

6g Protein
6g Fat
3g SatFat
0g Fibre
10g Carbs
116 Cals
0 5-a-day

Cappuccino *(skimmed)*
355ml, 12 fl oz, medium

7g Protein
0g Fat
0g SatFat
0g Fibre
11g Carbs
70 Cals
0 5-a-day

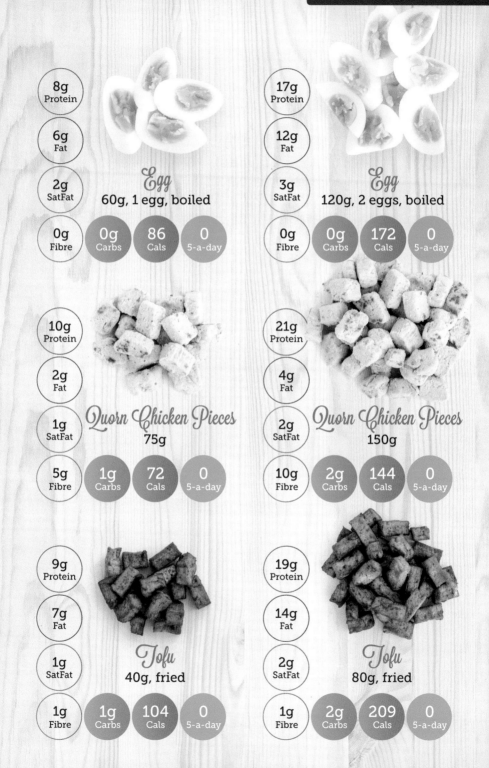

8g Protein
6g Fat
2g SatFat
0g Fibre

Egg
60g, 1 egg, boiled

0g Carbs | **86** Cals | **0** 5-a-day

17g Protein
12g Fat
3g SatFat
0g Fibre

Egg
120g, 2 eggs, boiled

0g Carbs | **172** Cals | **0** 5-a-day

10g Protein
2g Fat
1g SatFat
5g Fibre

Quorn Chicken Pieces
75g

1g Carbs | **72** Cals | **0** 5-a-day

21g Protein
4g Fat
2g SatFat
10g Fibre

Quorn Chicken Pieces
150g

2g Carbs | **144** Cals | **0** 5-a-day

9g Protein
7g Fat
1g SatFat
1g Fibre

Tofu
40g, fried

1g Carbs | **104** Cals | **0** 5-a-day

19g Protein
14g Fat
2g SatFat
1g Fibre

Tofu
80g, fried

2g Carbs | **209** Cals | **0** 5-a-day

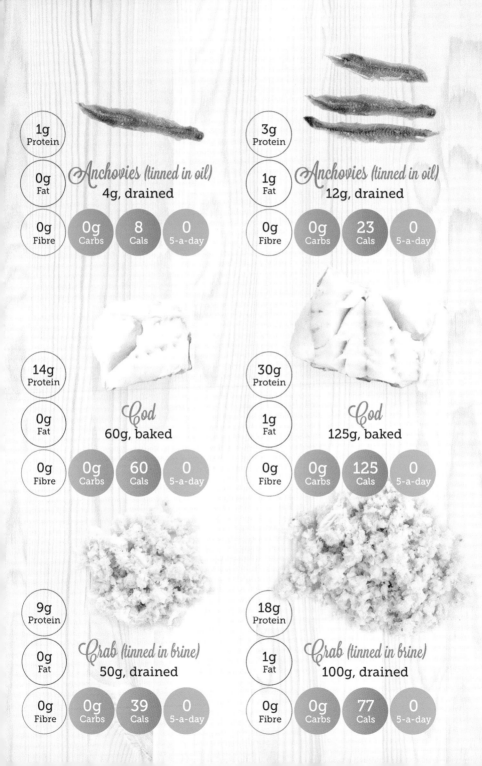

1g Protein
0g Fat
0g Fibre

Anchovies (tinned in oil)
4g, drained

0g Carbs
8 Cals
0 5-a-day

3g Protein
1g Fat
0g Fibre

Anchovies (tinned in oil)
12g, drained

0g Carbs
23 Cals
0 5-a-day

14g Protein
0g Fat
0g Fibre

Cod
60g, baked

0g Carbs
60 Cals
0 5-a-day

30g Protein
1g Fat
0g Fibre

Cod
125g, baked

0g Carbs
125 Cals
0 5-a-day

9g Protein
0g Fat
0g Fibre

Crab (tinned in brine)
50g, drained

0g Carbs
39 Cals
0 5-a-day

18g Protein
1g Fat
0g Fibre

Crab (tinned in brine)
100g, drained

0g Carbs
77 Cals
0 5-a-day

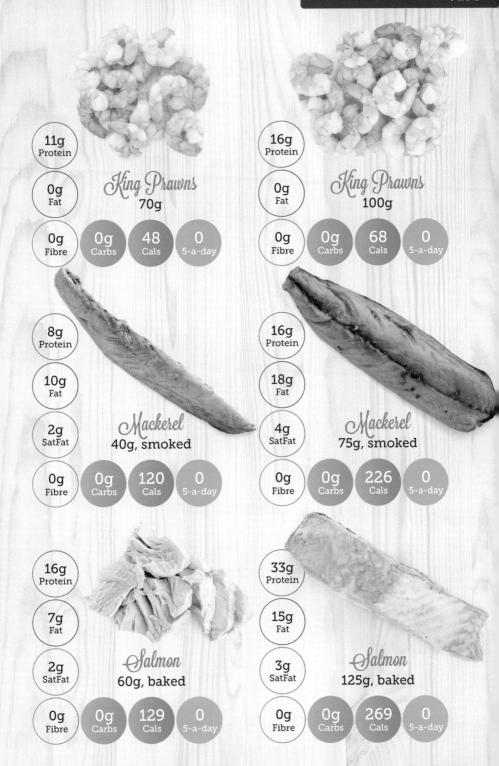

11g Protein

0g Fat

0g Fibre

King Prawns
70g

0g Carbs

48 Cals

0 5-a-day

16g Protein

0g Fat

0g Fibre

King Prawns
100g

0g Carbs

68 Cals

0 5-a-day

8g Protein

10g Fat

2g SatFat

0g Fibre

Mackerel
40g, smoked

0g Carbs

120 Cals

0 5-a-day

16g Protein

18g Fat

4g SatFat

0g Fibre

Mackerel
75g, smoked

0g Carbs

226 Cals

0 5-a-day

16g Protein

7g Fat

2g SatFat

0g Fibre

Salmon
60g, baked

0g Carbs

129 Cals

0 5-a-day

33g Protein

15g Fat

3g SatFat

0g Fibre

Salmon
125g, baked

0g Carbs

269 Cals

0 5-a-day

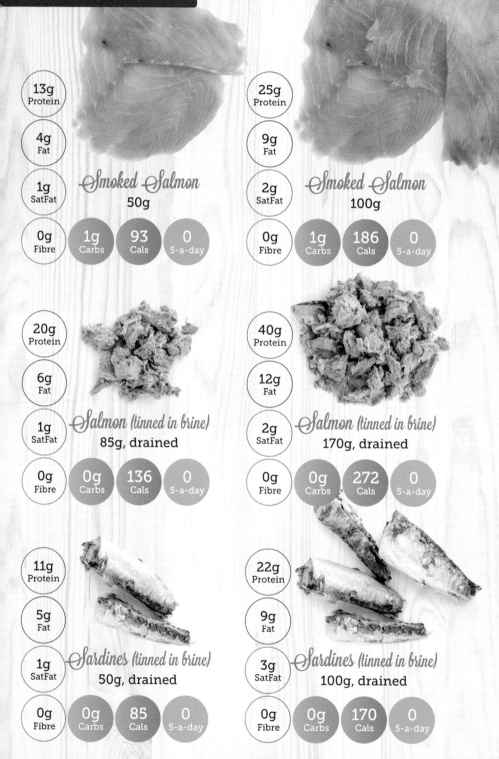

Smoked Salmon
50g

13g Protein
4g Fat
1g SatFat
0g Fibre
1g Carbs
93 Cals
0 5-a-day

Smoked Salmon
100g

25g Protein
9g Fat
2g SatFat
0g Fibre
1g Carbs
186 Cals
0 5-a-day

Salmon (tinned in brine)
85g, drained

20g Protein
6g Fat
1g SatFat
0g Fibre
0g Carbs
136 Cals
0 5-a-day

Salmon (tinned in brine)
170g, drained

40g Protein
12g Fat
2g SatFat
0g Fibre
0g Carbs
272 Cals
0 5-a-day

Sardines (tinned in brine)
50g, drained

11g Protein
5g Fat
1g SatFat
0g Fibre
0g Carbs
85 Cals
0 5-a-day

Sardines (tinned in brine)
100g, drained

22g Protein
9g Fat
3g SatFat
0g Fibre
0g Carbs
170 Cals
0 5-a-day

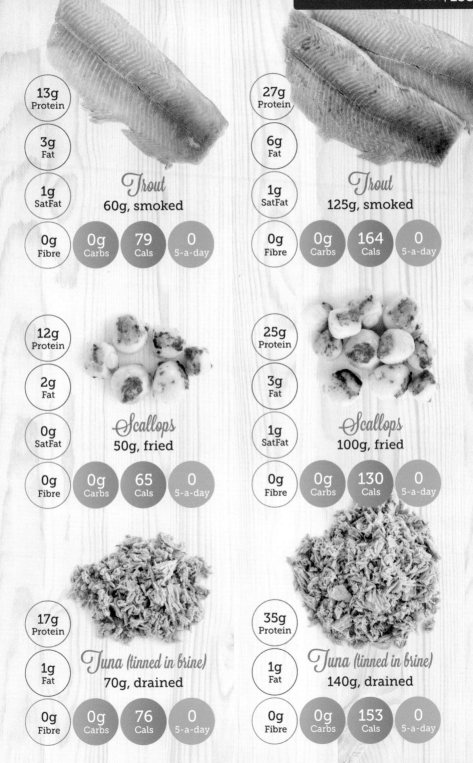

13g Protein
3g Fat
1g SatFat
0g Fibre
0g Carbs
79 Cals
0 5-a-day

Trout
60g, smoked

27g Protein
6g Fat
1g SatFat
0g Fibre
0g Carbs
164 Cals
0 5-a-day

Trout
125g, smoked

12g Protein
2g Fat
0g SatFat
0g Fibre
0g Carbs
65 Cals
0 5-a-day

Scallops
50g, fried

25g Protein
3g Fat
1g SatFat
0g Fibre
0g Carbs
130 Cals
0 5-a-day

Scallops
100g, fried

17g Protein
1g Fat
0g Fibre
0g Carbs
76 Cals
0 5-a-day

Tuna (tinned in brine)
70g, drained

35g Protein
1g Fat
0g Fibre
0g Carbs
153 Cals
0 5-a-day

Tuna (tinned in brine)
140g, drained

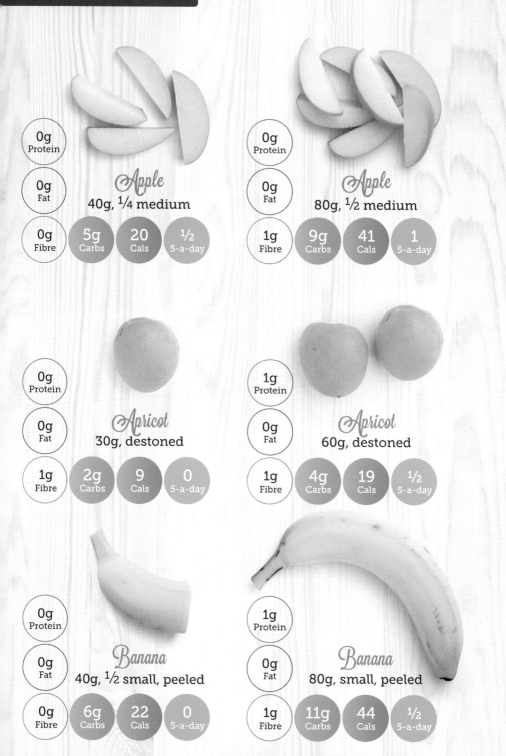

0g Protein			
0g Fat			
0g Fibre	5g Carbs	20 Cals	½ 5-a-day

Apple
40g, ¼ medium

0g Protein			
0g Fat			
1g Fibre	9g Carbs	41 Cals	1 5-a-day

Apple
80g, ½ medium

0g Protein			
0g Fat			
1g Fibre	2g Carbs	9 Cals	0 5-a-day

Apricot
30g, destoned

1g Protein			
0g Fat			
1g Fibre	4g Carbs	19 Cals	½ 5-a-day

Apricot
60g, destoned

0g Protein			
0g Fat			
0g Fibre	6g Carbs	22 Cals	0 5-a-day

Banana
40g, ½ small, peeled

1g Protein			
0g Fat			
1g Fibre	11g Carbs	44 Cals	½ 5-a-day

Banana
80g, small, peeled

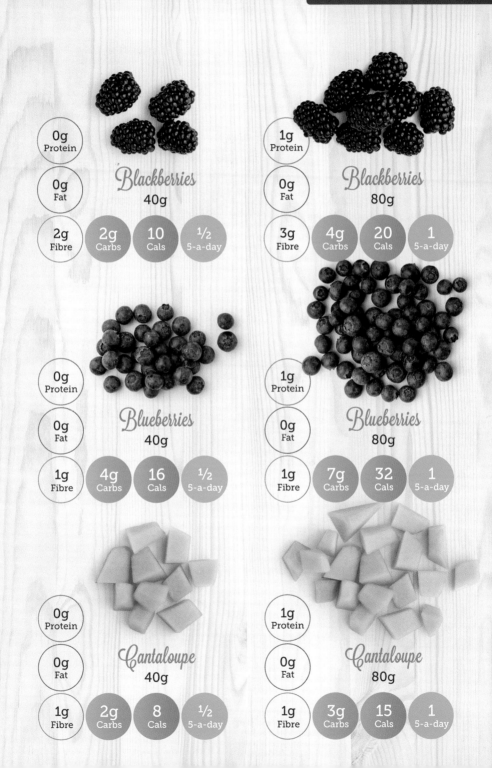

0g
Protein

0g
Fat

2g
Fibre

Blackberries
40g

2g
Carbs

10
Cals

½
5-a-day

1g
Protein

0g
Fat

3g
Fibre

Blackberries
80g

4g
Carbs

20
Cals

1
5-a-day

0g
Protein

0g
Fat

1g
Fibre

Blueberries
40g

4g
Carbs

16
Cals

½
5-a-day

1g
Protein

0g
Fat

1g
Fibre

Blueberries
80g

7g
Carbs

32
Cals

1
5-a-day

0g
Protein

0g
Fat

1g
Fibre

Cantaloupe
40g

2g
Carbs

8
Cals

½
5-a-day

1g
Protein

0g
Fat

1g
Fibre

Cantaloupe
80g

3g
Carbs

15
Cals

1
5-a-day

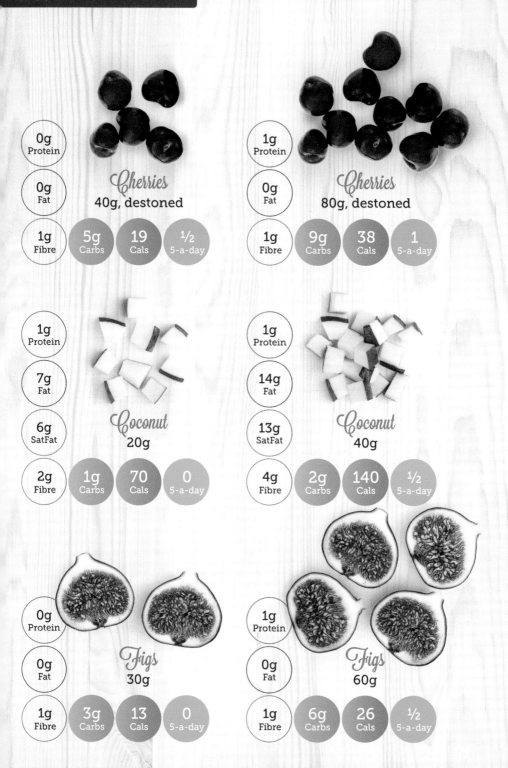

0g
Protein

0g
Fat

1g
Fibre

Cherries
40g, destoned

5g
Carbs

19
Cals

½
5-a-day

1g
Protein

0g
Fat

1g
Fibre

Cherries
80g, destoned

9g
Carbs

38
Cals

1
5-a-day

1g
Protein

7g
Fat

6g
SatFat

2g
Fibre

Coconut
20g

1g
Carbs

70
Cals

0
5-a-day

1g
Protein

14g
Fat

13g
SatFat

4g
Fibre

Coconut
40g

2g
Carbs

140
Cals

½
5-a-day

0g
Protein

0g
Fat

1g
Fibre

Figs
30g

3g
Carbs

13
Cals

0
5-a-day

1g
Protein

0g
Fat

1g
Fibre

Figs
60g

6g
Carbs

26
Cals

½
5-a-day

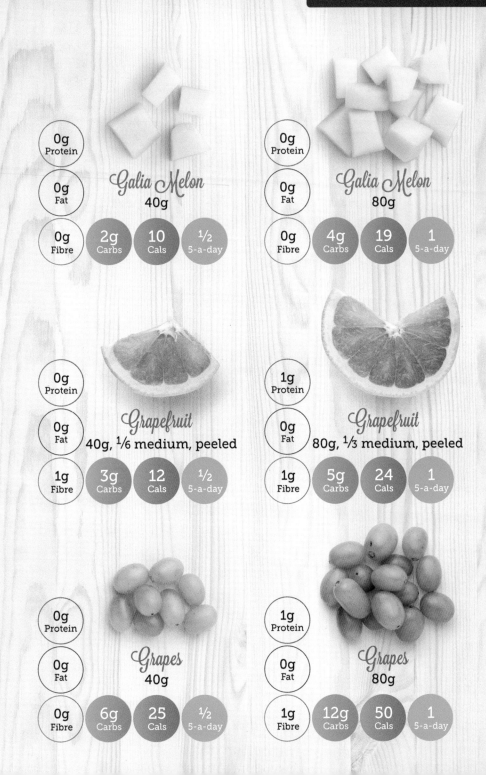

0g Protein
0g Fat
0g Fibre

Galia Melon
40g

2g Carbs
10 Cals
½ 5-a-day

0g Protein
0g Fat
0g Fibre

Galia Melon
80g

4g Carbs
19 Cals
1 5-a-day

0g Protein
0g Fat
1g Fibre

Grapefruit
40g, ⅙ medium, peeled

3g Carbs
12 Cals
½ 5-a-day

1g Protein
0g Fat
1g Fibre

Grapefruit
80g, ⅓ medium, peeled

5g Carbs
24 Cals
1 5-a-day

0g Protein
0g Fat
0g Fibre

Grapes
40g

6g Carbs
25 Cals
½ 5-a-day

1g Protein
0g Fat
1g Fibre

Grapes
80g

12g Carbs
50 Cals
1 5-a-day

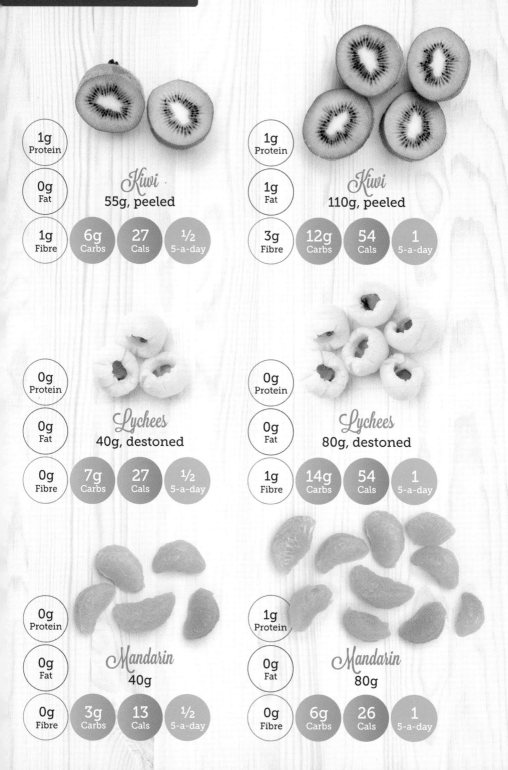

1g Protein

0g Fat

1g Fibre

Kiwi
55g, peeled

6g Carbs

27 Cals

½ 5-a-day

1g Protein

1g Fat

3g Fibre

Kiwi
110g, peeled

12g Carbs

54 Cals

1 5-a-day

0g Protein

0g Fat

0g Fibre

Lychees
40g, destoned

7g Carbs

27 Cals

½ 5-a-day

0g Protein

0g Fat

1g Fibre

Lychees
80g, destoned

14g Carbs

54 Cals

1 5-a-day

0g Protein

0g Fat

0g Fibre

Mandarin
40g

3g Carbs

13 Cals

½ 5-a-day

1g Protein

0g Fat

0g Fibre

Mandarin
80g

6g Carbs

26 Cals

1 5-a-day

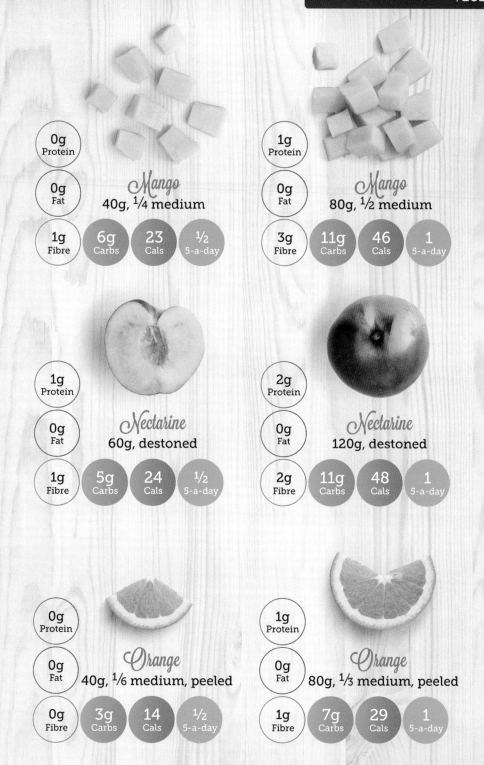

0g Protein

0g Fat

1g Fibre

Mango
40g, ¼ medium

6g Carbs | **23** Cals | **½** 5-a-day

1g Protein

0g Fat

3g Fibre

Mango
80g, ½ medium

11g Carbs | **46** Cals | **1** 5-a-day

1g Protein

0g Fat

1g Fibre

Nectarine
60g, destoned

5g Carbs | **24** Cals | **½** 5-a-day

2g Protein

0g Fat

2g Fibre

Nectarine
120g, destoned

11g Carbs | **48** Cals | **1** 5-a-day

0g Protein

0g Fat

0g Fibre

Orange
40g, ⅙ medium, peeled

3g Carbs | **14** Cals | **½** 5-a-day

1g Protein

0g Fat

1g Fibre

Orange
80g, ⅓ medium, peeled

7g Carbs | **29** Cals | **1** 5-a-day

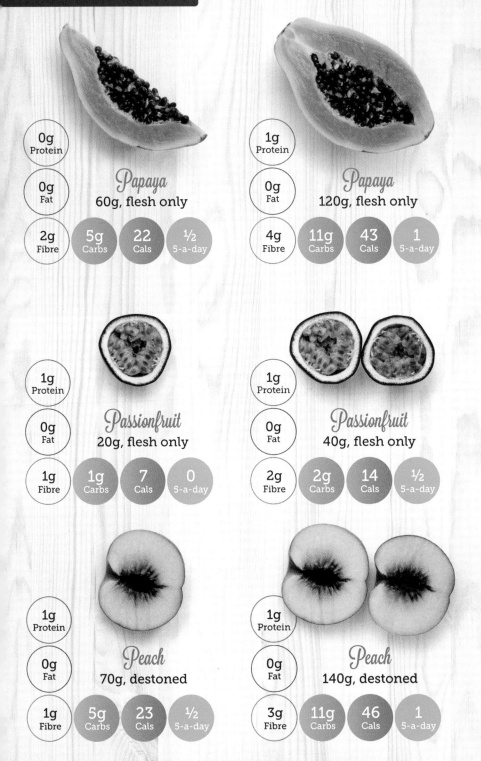

Papaya
60g, flesh only

0g Protein
0g Fat
2g Fibre
5g Carbs
22 Cals
½ 5-a-day

Papaya
120g, flesh only

1g Protein
0g Fat
4g Fibre
11g Carbs
43 Cals
1 5-a-day

Passionfruit
20g, flesh only

1g Protein
0g Fat
1g Fibre
1g Carbs
7 Cals
0 5-a-day

Passionfruit
40g, flesh only

1g Protein
0g Fat
2g Fibre
2g Carbs
14 Cals
½ 5-a-day

Peach
70g, destoned

1g Protein
0g Fat
1g Fibre
5g Carbs
23 Cals
½ 5-a-day

Peach
140g, destoned

1g Protein
0g Fat
3g Fibre
11g Carbs
46 Cals
1 5-a-day

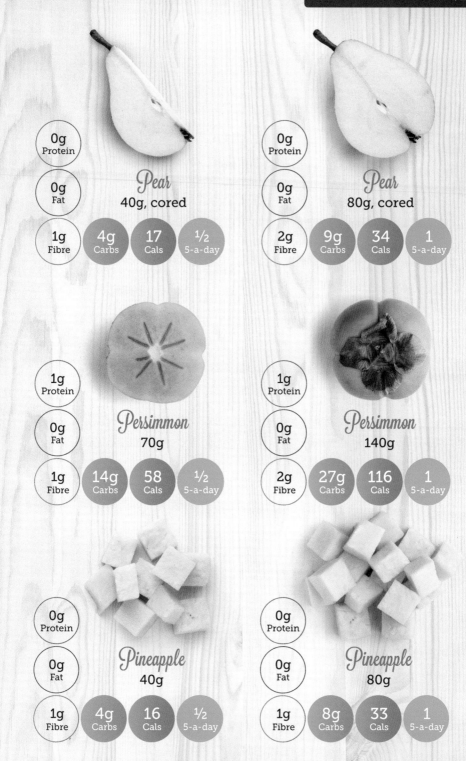

0g
Protein

0g
Fat

Pear
40g, cored

1g
Fibre

4g
Carbs

17
Cals

½
5-a-day

0g
Protein

0g
Fat

Pear
80g, cored

2g
Fibre

9g
Carbs

34
Cals

1
5-a-day

1g
Protein

0g
Fat

Persimmon
70g

1g
Fibre

14g
Carbs

58
Cals

½
5-a-day

1g
Protein

0g
Fat

Persimmon
140g

2g
Fibre

27g
Carbs

116
Cals

1
5-a-day

0g
Protein

0g
Fat

Pineapple
40g

1g
Fibre

4g
Carbs

16
Cals

½
5-a-day

0g
Protein

0g
Fat

Pineapple
80g

1g
Fibre

8g
Carbs

33
Cals

1
5-a-day

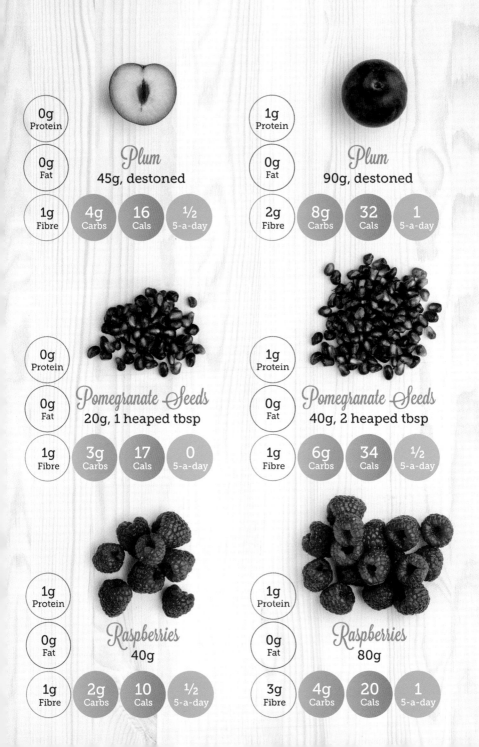

0g Protein
0g Fat
1g Fibre
Plum
45g, destoned
4g Carbs
16 Cals
½ 5-a-day

1g Protein
0g Fat
2g Fibre
Plum
90g, destoned
8g Carbs
32 Cals
1 5-a-day

0g Protein
0g Fat
1g Fibre
Pomegranate Seeds
20g, 1 heaped tbsp
3g Carbs
17 Cals
0 5-a-day

1g Protein
0g Fat
1g Fibre
Pomegranate Seeds
40g, 2 heaped tbsp
6g Carbs
34 Cals
½ 5-a-day

1g Protein
0g Fat
1g Fibre
Raspberries
40g
2g Carbs
10 Cals
½ 5-a-day

1g Protein
0g Fat
3g Fibre
Raspberries
80g
4g Carbs
20 Cals
1 5-a-day

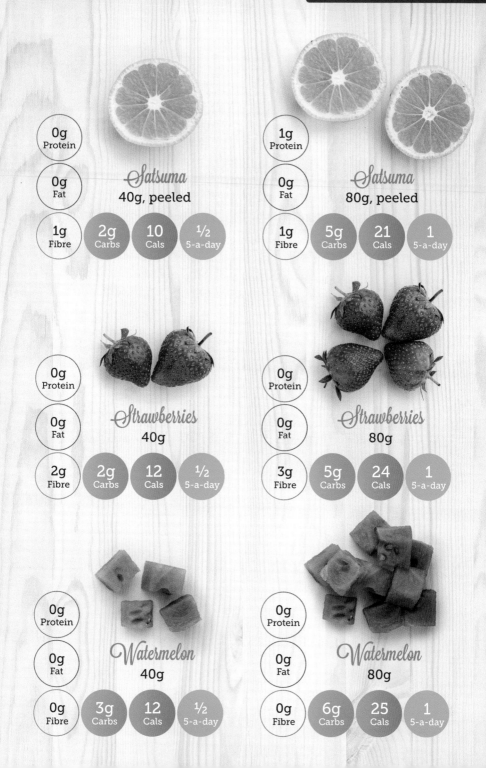

0g
Protein

0g
Fat

1g
Fibre

Satsuma
40g, peeled

2g
Carbs

10
Cals

½
5-a-day

1g
Protein

0g
Fat

1g
Fibre

Satsuma
80g, peeled

5g
Carbs

21
Cals

1
5-a-day

0g
Protein

0g
Fat

2g
Fibre

Strawberries
40g

2g
Carbs

12
Cals

½
5-a-day

0g
Protein

0g
Fat

3g
Fibre

Strawberries
80g

5g
Carbs

24
Cals

1
5-a-day

0g
Protein

0g
Fat

0g
Fibre

Watermelon
40g

3g
Carbs

12
Cals

½
5-a-day

0g
Protein

0g
Fat

0g
Fibre

Watermelon
80g

6g
Carbs

25
Cals

1
5-a-day

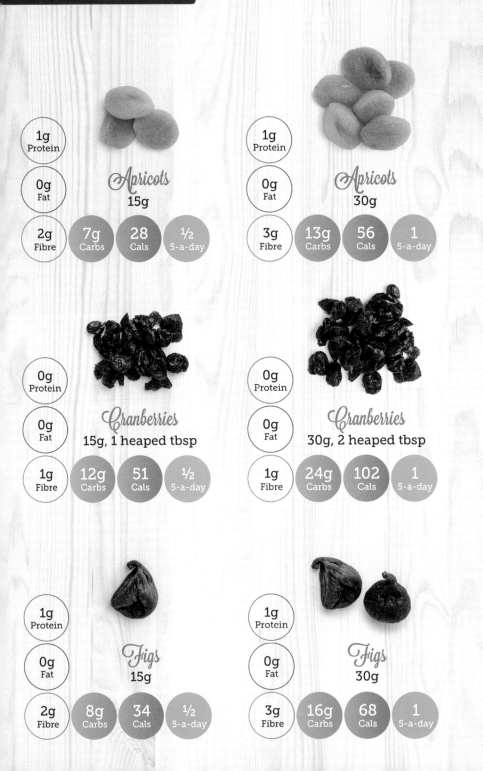

Apricots
15g

1g Protein
0g Fat
2g Fibre
7g Carbs
28 Cals
½ 5-a-day

Apricots
30g

1g Protein
0g Fat
3g Fibre
13g Carbs
56 Cals
1 5-a-day

Cranberries
15g, 1 heaped tbsp

0g Protein
0g Fat
1g Fibre
12g Carbs
51 Cals
½ 5-a-day

Cranberries
30g, 2 heaped tbsp

0g Protein
0g Fat
1g Fibre
24g Carbs
102 Cals
1 5-a-day

Figs
15g

1g Protein
0g Fat
2g Fibre
8g Carbs
34 Cals
½ 5-a-day

Figs
30g

1g Protein
0g Fat
3g Fibre
16g Carbs
68 Cals
1 5-a-day

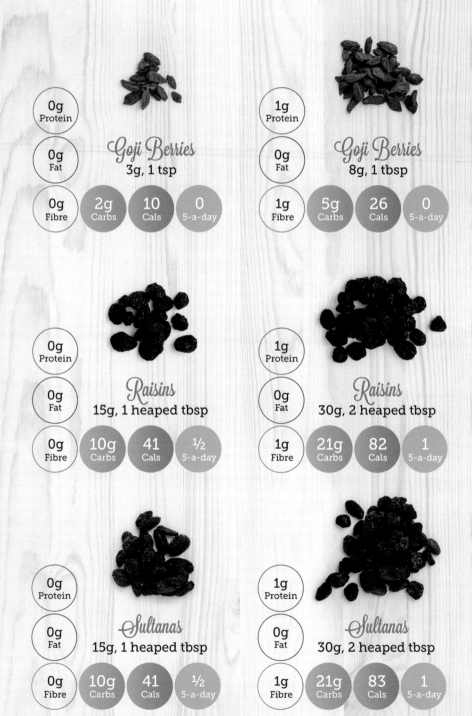

0g Protein

0g Fat

0g Fibre

Goji Berries
3g, 1 tsp

2g Carbs

10 Cals

0 5-a-day

1g Protein

0g Fat

1g Fibre

Goji Berries
8g, 1 tbsp

5g Carbs

26 Cals

0 5-a-day

0g Protein

0g Fat

0g Fibre

Raisins
15g, 1 heaped tbsp

10g Carbs

41 Cals

½ 5-a-day

1g Protein

0g Fat

1g Fibre

Raisins
30g, 2 heaped tbsp

21g Carbs

82 Cals

1 5-a-day

0g Protein

0g Fat

0g Fibre

Sultanas
15g, 1 heaped tbsp

10g Carbs

41 Cals

½ 5-a-day

1g Protein

0g Fat

1g Fibre

Sultanas
30g, 2 heaped tbsp

21g Carbs

83 Cals

1 5-a-day

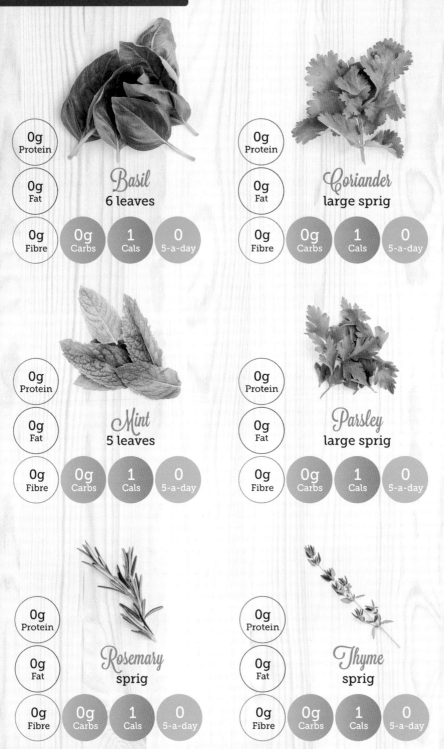

Basil
6 leaves

- 0g Protein
- 0g Fat
- 0g Fibre
- 0g Carbs
- 1 Cals
- 0 5-a-day

Coriander
large sprig

- 0g Protein
- 0g Fat
- 0g Fibre
- 0g Carbs
- 1 Cals
- 0 5-a-day

Mint
5 leaves

- 0g Protein
- 0g Fat
- 0g Fibre
- 0g Carbs
- 1 Cals
- 0 5-a-day

Parsley
large sprig

- 0g Protein
- 0g Fat
- 0g Fibre
- 0g Carbs
- 1 Cals
- 0 5-a-day

Rosemary
sprig

- 0g Protein
- 0g Fat
- 0g Fibre
- 0g Carbs
- 1 Cals
- 0 5-a-day

Thyme
sprig

- 0g Protein
- 0g Fat
- 0g Fibre
- 0g Carbs
- 1 Cals
- 0 5-a-day

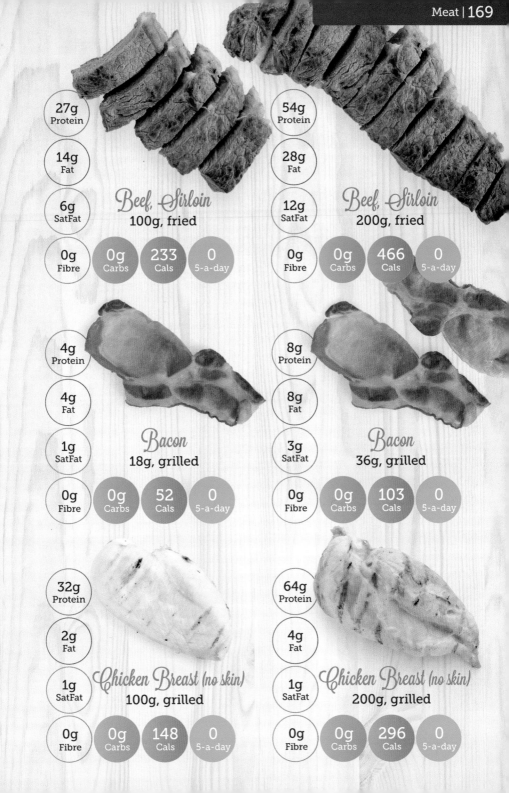

27g Protein
14g Fat
6g SatFat
0g Fibre
0g Carbs
233 Cals
0 5-a-day

Beef, Sirloin
100g, fried

54g Protein
28g Fat
12g SatFat
0g Fibre
0g Carbs
466 Cals
0 5-a-day

Beef, Sirloin
200g, fried

4g Protein
4g Fat
1g SatFat
0g Fibre
0g Carbs
52 Cals
0 5-a-day

Bacon
18g, grilled

8g Protein
8g Fat
3g SatFat
0g Fibre
0g Carbs
103 Cals
0 5-a-day

Bacon
36g, grilled

32g Protein
2g Fat
1g SatFat
0g Fibre
0g Carbs
148 Cals
0 5-a-day

Chicken Breast (no skin)
100g, grilled

64g Protein
4g Fat
1g SatFat
0g Fibre
0g Carbs
296 Cals
0 5-a-day

Chicken Breast (no skin)
200g, grilled

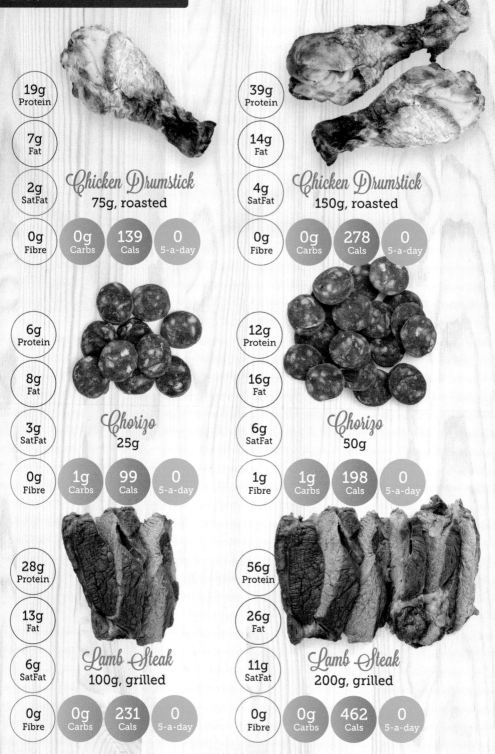

19g Protein
7g Fat
2g SatFat
0g Fibre

Chicken Drumstick
75g, roasted

0g Carbs | 139 Cals | 0 5-a-day

39g Protein
14g Fat
4g SatFat
0g Fibre

Chicken Drumstick
150g, roasted

0g Carbs | 278 Cals | 0 5-a-day

6g Protein
8g Fat
3g SatFat
0g Fibre

Chorizo
25g

1g Carbs | 99 Cals | 0 5-a-day

12g Protein
16g Fat
6g SatFat
1g Fibre

Chorizo
50g

1g Carbs | 198 Cals | 0 5-a-day

28g Protein
13g Fat
6g SatFat
0g Fibre

Lamb Steak
100g, grilled

0g Carbs | 231 Cals | 0 5-a-day

56g Protein
26g Fat
11g SatFat
0g Fibre

Lamb Steak
200g, grilled

0g Carbs | 462 Cals | 0 5-a-day

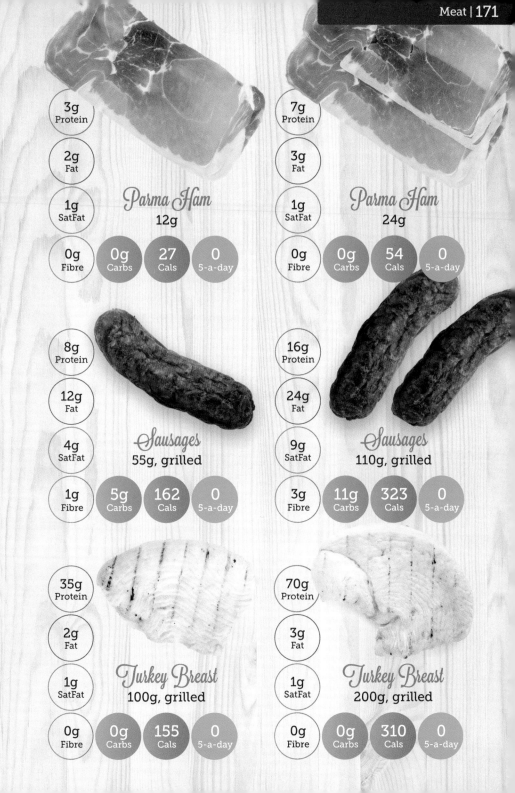

3g
Protein

2g
Fat

1g
SatFat

0g
Fibre

Parma Ham
12g

0g
Carbs

27
Cals

0
5-a-day

7g
Protein

3g
Fat

1g
SatFat

0g
Fibre

Parma Ham
24g

0g
Carbs

54
Cals

0
5-a-day

8g
Protein

12g
Fat

4g
SatFat

1g
Fibre

Sausages
55g, grilled

5g
Carbs

162
Cals

0
5-a-day

16g
Protein

24g
Fat

9g
SatFat

3g
Fibre

Sausages
110g, grilled

11g
Carbs

323
Cals

0
5-a-day

35g
Protein

2g
Fat

1g
SatFat

0g
Fibre

Turkey Breast
100g, grilled

0g
Carbs

155
Cals

0
5-a-day

70g
Protein

3g
Fat

1g
SatFat

0g
Fibre

Turkey Breast
200g, grilled

0g
Carbs

310
Cals

0
5-a-day

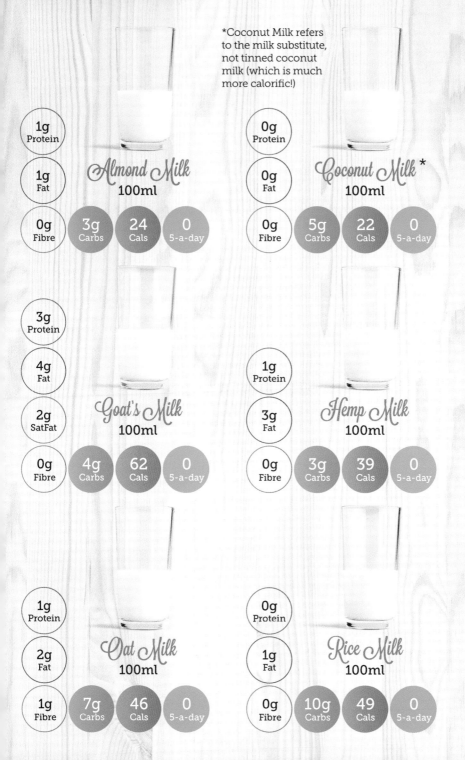

*Coconut Milk refers to the milk substitute, not tinned coconut milk (which is much more calorific!)

Almond Milk
100ml

- 1g Protein
- 1g Fat
- 0g Fibre
- 3g Carbs
- 24 Cals
- 0 5-a-day

Coconut Milk *
100ml

- 0g Protein
- 0g Fat
- 0g Fibre
- 5g Carbs
- 22 Cals
- 0 5-a-day

Goat's Milk
100ml

- 3g Protein
- 4g Fat
- 2g SatFat
- 0g Fibre
- 4g Carbs
- 62 Cals
- 0 5-a-day

Hemp Milk
100ml

- 1g Protein
- 3g Fat
- 0g Fibre
- 3g Carbs
- 39 Cals
- 0 5-a-day

Oat Milk
100ml

- 1g Protein
- 2g Fat
- 1g Fibre
- 7g Carbs
- 46 Cals
- 0 5-a-day

Rice Milk
100ml

- 0g Protein
- 1g Fat
- 0g Fibre
- 10g Carbs
- 49 Cals
- 0 5-a-day

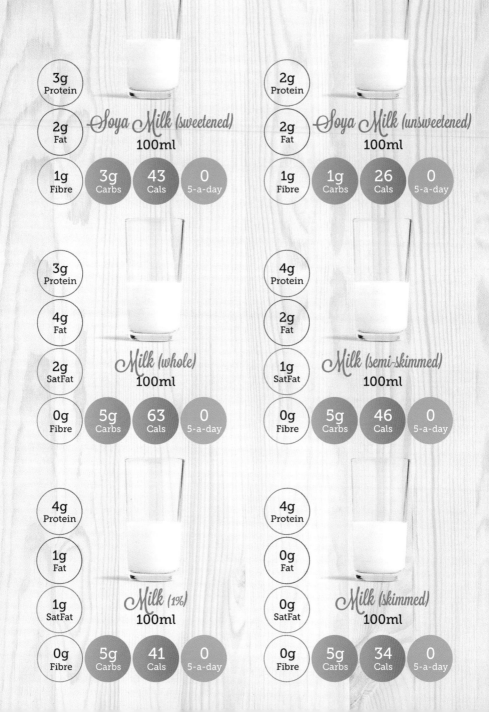

3g Protein
2g Fat
1g Fibre
Soya Milk (sweetened)
100ml
3g Carbs
43 Cals
0 5-a-day

2g Protein
2g Fat
1g Fibre
Soya Milk (unsweetened)
100ml
1g Carbs
26 Cals
0 5-a-day

3g Protein
4g Fat
2g SatFat
0g Fibre
Milk (whole)
100ml
5g Carbs
63 Cals
0 5-a-day

4g Protein
2g Fat
1g SatFat
0g Fibre
Milk (semi-skimmed)
100ml
5g Carbs
46 Cals
0 5-a-day

4g Protein
1g Fat
1g SatFat
0g Fibre
Milk (1%)
100ml
5g Carbs
41 Cals
0 5-a-day

4g Protein
0g Fat
0g SatFat
0g Fibre
Milk (skimmed)
100ml
5g Carbs
34 Cals
0 5-a-day

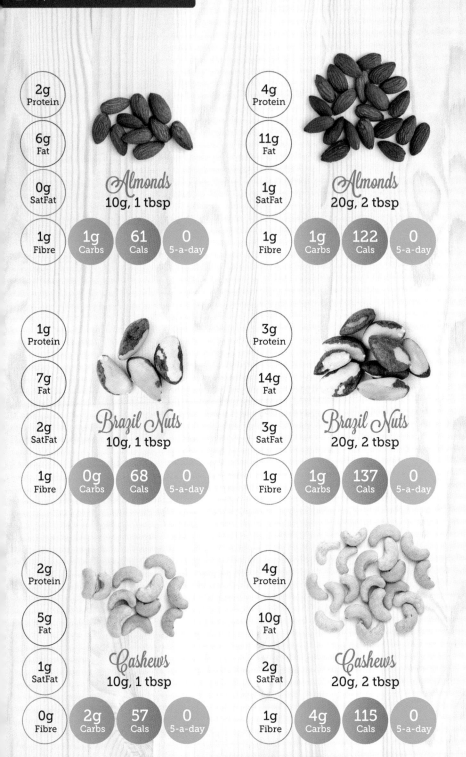

Almonds
10g, 1 tbsp

- 2g Protein
- 6g Fat
- 0g SatFat
- 1g Fibre
- 1g Carbs
- 61 Cals
- 0 5-a-day

Almonds
20g, 2 tbsp

- 4g Protein
- 11g Fat
- 1g SatFat
- 1g Fibre
- 1g Carbs
- 122 Cals
- 0 5-a-day

Brazil Nuts
10g, 1 tbsp

- 1g Protein
- 7g Fat
- 2g SatFat
- 1g Fibre
- 0g Carbs
- 68 Cals
- 0 5-a-day

Brazil Nuts
20g, 2 tbsp

- 3g Protein
- 14g Fat
- 3g SatFat
- 1g Fibre
- 1g Carbs
- 137 Cals
- 0 5-a-day

Cashews
10g, 1 tbsp

- 2g Protein
- 5g Fat
- 1g SatFat
- 0g Fibre
- 2g Carbs
- 57 Cals
- 0 5-a-day

Cashews
20g, 2 tbsp

- 4g Protein
- 10g Fat
- 2g SatFat
- 1g Fibre
- 4g Carbs
- 115 Cals
- 0 5-a-day

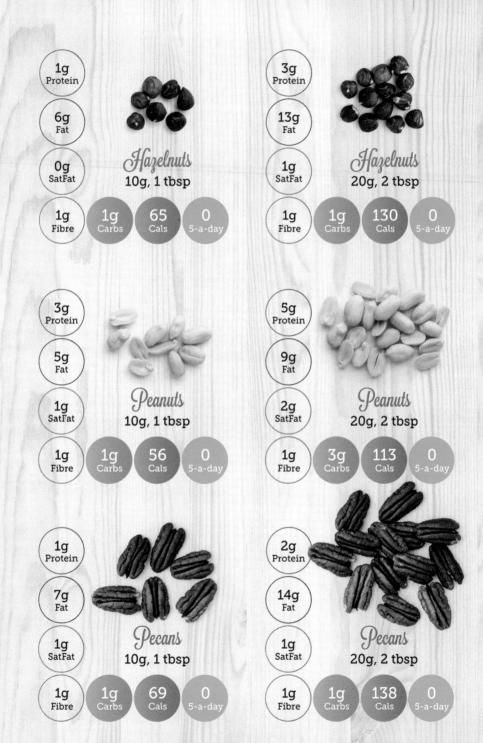

1g Protein
6g Fat
0g SatFat
1g Fibre

Hazelnuts
10g, 1 tbsp

1g Carbs | 65 Cals | 0 5-a-day

3g Protein
13g Fat
1g SatFat
1g Fibre

Hazelnuts
20g, 2 tbsp

1g Carbs | 130 Cals | 0 5-a-day

3g Protein
5g Fat
1g SatFat
1g Fibre

Peanuts
10g, 1 tbsp

1g Carbs | 56 Cals | 0 5-a-day

5g Protein
9g Fat
2g SatFat
1g Fibre

Peanuts
20g, 2 tbsp

3g Carbs | 113 Cals | 0 5-a-day

1g Protein
7g Fat
1g SatFat
1g Fibre

Pecans
10g, 1 tbsp

1g Carbs | 69 Cals | 0 5-a-day

2g Protein
14g Fat
1g SatFat
1g Fibre

Pecans
20g, 2 tbsp

1g Carbs | 138 Cals | 0 5-a-day

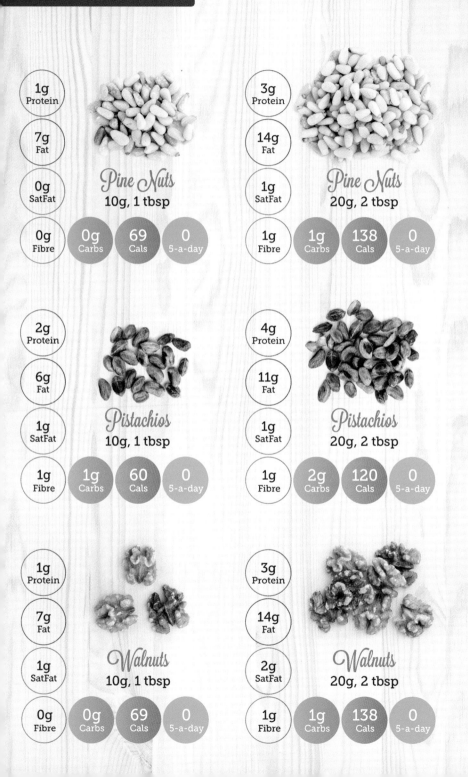

1g Protein
7g Fat
0g SatFat
0g Fibre

Pine Nuts
10g, 1 tbsp

0g Carbs | 69 Cals | 0 5-a-day

3g Protein
14g Fat
1g SatFat
1g Fibre

Pine Nuts
20g, 2 tbsp

1g Carbs | 138 Cals | 0 5-a-day

2g Protein
6g Fat
1g SatFat
1g Fibre

Pistachios
10g, 1 tbsp

1g Carbs | 60 Cals | 0 5-a-day

4g Protein
11g Fat
1g SatFat
1g Fibre

Pistachios
20g, 2 tbsp

2g Carbs | 120 Cals | 0 5-a-day

1g Protein
7g Fat
1g SatFat
0g Fibre

Walnuts
10g, 1 tbsp

0g Carbs | 69 Cals | 0 5-a-day

3g Protein
14g Fat
2g SatFat
1g Fibre

Walnuts
20g, 2 tbsp

1g Carbs | 138 Cals | 0 5-a-day

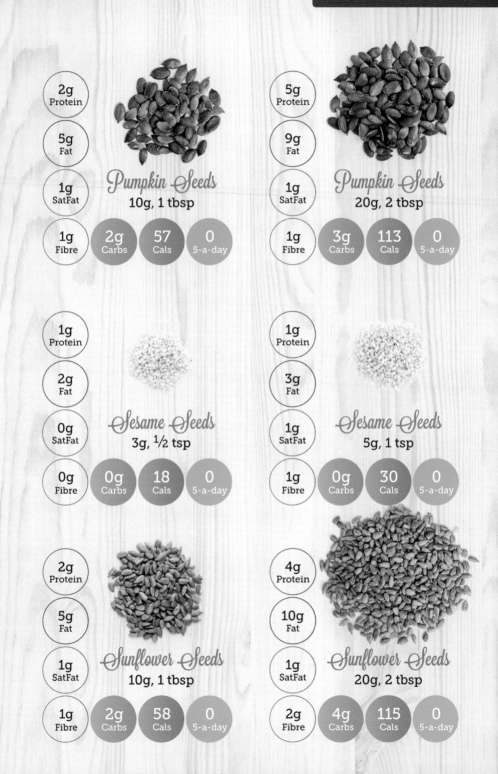

2g Protein
5g Fat
1g SatFat
1g Fibre
2g Carbs
57 Cals
0 5-a-day

Pumpkin Seeds
10g, 1 tbsp

5g Protein
9g Fat
1g SatFat
1g Fibre
3g Carbs
113 Cals
0 5-a-day

Pumpkin Seeds
20g, 2 tbsp

1g Protein
2g Fat
0g SatFat
0g Fibre
0g Carbs
18 Cals
0 5-a-day

Sesame Seeds
3g, ½ tsp

1g Protein
3g Fat
1g SatFat
1g Fibre
0g Carbs
30 Cals
0 5-a-day

Sesame Seeds
5g, 1 tsp

2g Protein
5g Fat
1g SatFat
1g Fibre
2g Carbs
58 Cals
0 5-a-day

Sunflower Seeds
10g, 1 tbsp

4g Protein
10g Fat
1g SatFat
2g Fibre
4g Carbs
115 Cals
0 5-a-day

Sunflower Seeds
20g, 2 tbsp

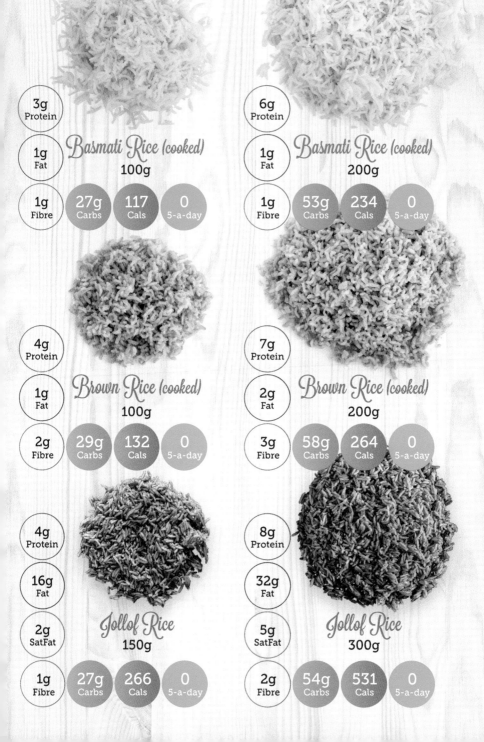

Basmati Rice (cooked)
100g

3g Protein
1g Fat
1g Fibre
27g Carbs
117 Cals
0 5-a-day

Basmati Rice (cooked)
200g

6g Protein
1g Fat
1g Fibre
53g Carbs
234 Cals
0 5-a-day

Brown Rice (cooked)
100g

4g Protein
1g Fat
2g Fibre
29g Carbs
132 Cals
0 5-a-day

Brown Rice (cooked)
200g

7g Protein
2g Fat
3g Fibre
58g Carbs
264 Cals
0 5-a-day

Jollof Rice
150g

4g Protein
16g Fat
2g SatFat
1g Fibre
27g Carbs
266 Cals
0 5-a-day

Jollof Rice
300g

8g Protein
32g Fat
5g SatFat
2g Fibre
54g Carbs
531 Cals
0 5-a-day

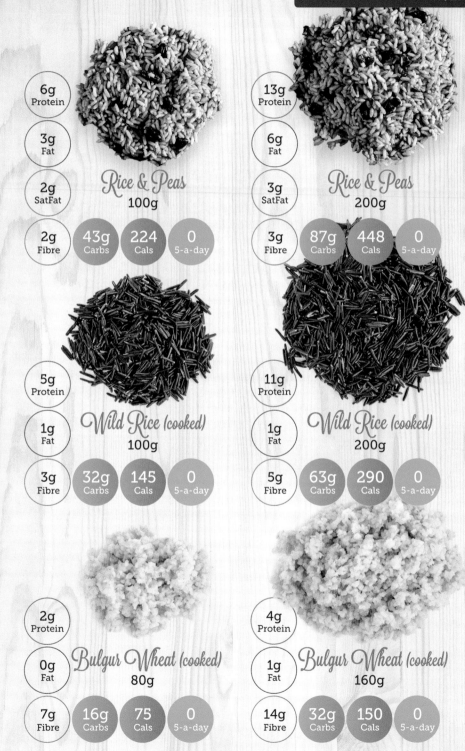

Rice & Peas
100g

- 6g Protein
- 3g Fat
- 2g SatFat
- 2g Fibre
- 43g Carbs
- 224 Cals
- 0 5-a-day

Rice & Peas
200g

- 13g Protein
- 6g Fat
- 3g SatFat
- 3g Fibre
- 87g Carbs
- 448 Cals
- 0 5-a-day

Wild Rice (cooked)
100g

- 5g Protein
- 1g Fat
- 3g Fibre
- 32g Carbs
- 145 Cals
- 0 5-a-day

Wild Rice (cooked)
200g

- 11g Protein
- 1g Fat
- 5g Fibre
- 63g Carbs
- 290 Cals
- 0 5-a-day

Bulgur Wheat (cooked)
80g

- 2g Protein
- 0g Fat
- 7g Fibre
- 16g Carbs
- 75 Cals
- 0 5-a-day

Bulgur Wheat (cooked)
160g

- 4g Protein
- 1g Fat
- 14g Fibre
- 32g Carbs
- 150 Cals
- 0 5-a-day

Couscous (cooked) 80g

- 6g Protein
- 1g Fat
- 2g Fibre
- 30g Carbs
- 142 Cals
- 0 5-a-day

Couscous (cooked) 160g

- 12g Protein
- 2g Fat
- 4g Fibre
- 60g Carbs
- 285 Cals
- 0 5-a-day

Pearl Barley (cooked) 80g

- 2g Protein
- 0g Fat
- 3g Fibre
- 22g Carbs
- 96 Cals
- 0 5-a-day

Pearl Barley (cooked) 160g

- 4g Protein
- 1g Fat
- 6g Fibre
- 44g Carbs
- 192 Cals
- 0 5-a-day

Quinoa (cooked) 80g

- 4g Protein
- 2g Fat
- 2g Fibre
- 15g Carbs
- 92 Cals
- 0 5-a-day

Quinoa (cooked) 160g

- 7g Protein
- 3g Fat
- 5g Fibre
- 30g Carbs
- 184 Cals
- 0 5-a-day

6g Protein

1g Fat

Egg Noodles (cooked)
100g

3g Fibre | **36g** Carbs | **166** Cals | **0** 5-a-day

12g Protein

2g Fat

Egg Noodles (cooked)
200g

6g Fibre | **71g** Carbs | **332** Cals | **0** 5-a-day

5g Protein

0g Fat

Pasta (cooked)
100g

3g Fibre | **33g** Carbs | **146** Cals | **0** 5-a-day

10g Protein

1g Fat

Pasta (cooked)
200g

5g Fibre | **66g** Carbs | **292** Cals | **0** 5-a-day

5g Protein

1g Fat

Pasta Wholewheat (cooked)
100g

4g Fibre | **28g** Carbs | **134** Cals | **0** 5-a-day

10g Protein

2g Fat

Pasta Wholewheat (cooked)
200g

8g Fibre | **55g** Carbs | **268** Cals | **0** 5-a-day

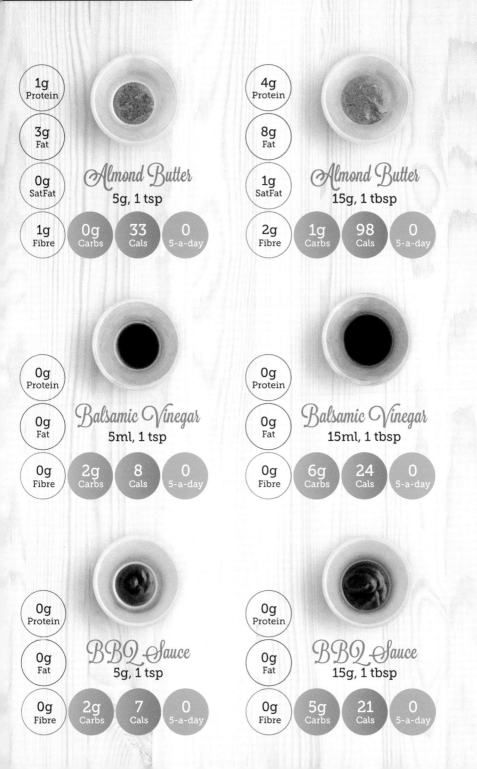

1g Protein
3g Fat
0g SatFat
1g Fibre
0g Carbs
33 Cals
0 5-a-day

Almond Butter
5g, 1 tsp

4g Protein
8g Fat
1g SatFat
2g Fibre
1g Carbs
98 Cals
0 5-a-day

Almond Butter
15g, 1 tbsp

0g Protein
0g Fat
0g Fibre
2g Carbs
8 Cals
0 5-a-day

Balsamic Vinegar
5ml, 1 tsp

0g Protein
0g Fat
0g Fibre
6g Carbs
24 Cals
0 5-a-day

Balsamic Vinegar
15ml, 1 tbsp

0g Protein
0g Fat
0g Fibre
2g Carbs
7 Cals
0 5-a-day

BBQ Sauce
5g, 1 tsp

0g Protein
0g Fat
0g Fibre
5g Carbs
21 Cals
0 5-a-day

BBQ Sauce
15g, 1 tbsp

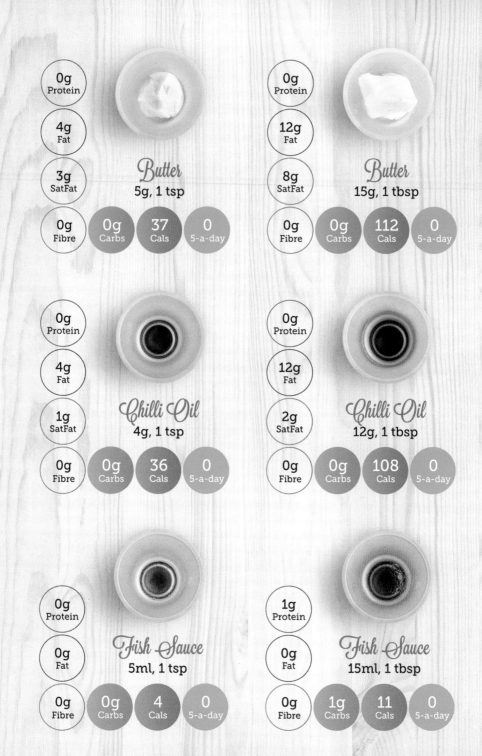

Butter
5g, 1 tsp

0g Protein
4g Fat
3g SatFat
0g Fibre
0g Carbs
37 Cals
0 5-a-day

Butter
15g, 1 tbsp

0g Protein
12g Fat
8g SatFat
0g Fibre
0g Carbs
112 Cals
0 5-a-day

Chilli Oil
4g, 1 tsp

0g Protein
4g Fat
1g SatFat
0g Fibre
0g Carbs
36 Cals
0 5-a-day

Chilli Oil
12g, 1 tbsp

0g Protein
12g Fat
2g SatFat
0g Fibre
0g Carbs
108 Cals
0 5-a-day

Fish Sauce
5ml, 1 tsp

0g Protein
0g Fat
0g Fibre
0g Carbs
4 Cals
0 5-a-day

Fish Sauce
15ml, 1 tbsp

1g Protein
0g Fat
0g Fibre
1g Carbs
11 Cals
0 5-a-day

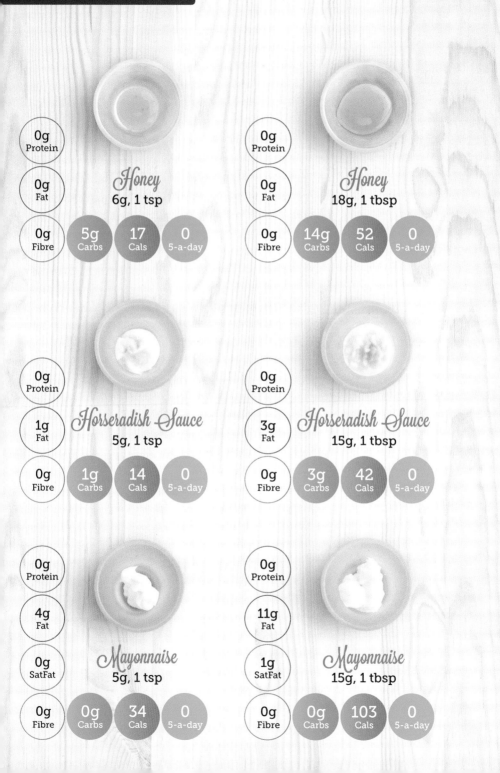

Honey
6g, 1 tsp

0g Protein
0g Fat
0g Fibre
5g Carbs
17 Cals
0 5-a-day

Honey
18g, 1 tbsp

0g Protein
0g Fat
0g Fibre
14g Carbs
52 Cals
0 5-a-day

Horseradish Sauce
5g, 1 tsp

0g Protein
1g Fat
0g Fibre
1g Carbs
14 Cals
0 5-a-day

Horseradish Sauce
15g, 1 tbsp

0g Protein
3g Fat
0g Fibre
3g Carbs
42 Cals
0 5-a-day

Mayonnaise
5g, 1 tsp

0g Protein
4g Fat
0g SatFat
0g Fibre
0g Carbs
34 Cals
0 5-a-day

Mayonnaise
15g, 1 tbsp

0g Protein
11g Fat
1g SatFat
0g Fibre
0g Carbs
103 Cals
0 5-a-day

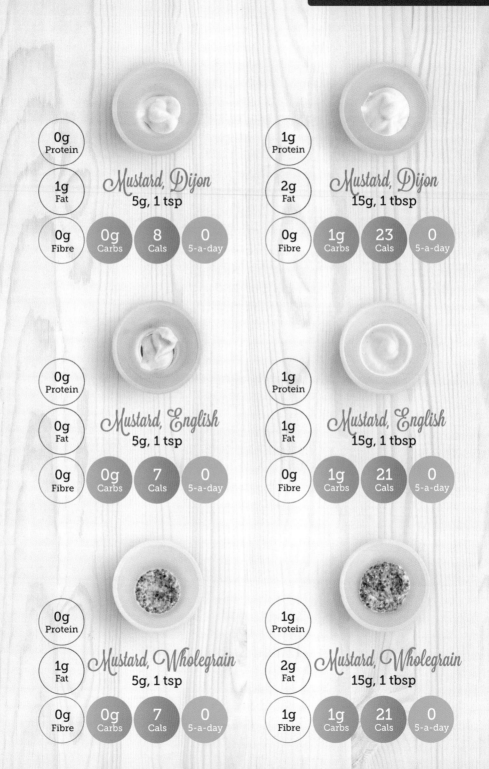

Mustard, Dijon
5g, 1 tsp

- 0g Protein
- 1g Fat
- 0g Fibre
- 0g Carbs
- 8 Cals
- 0 5-a-day

Mustard, Dijon
15g, 1 tbsp

- 1g Protein
- 2g Fat
- 0g Fibre
- 1g Carbs
- 23 Cals
- 0 5-a-day

Mustard, English
5g, 1 tsp

- 0g Protein
- 0g Fat
- 0g Fibre
- 0g Carbs
- 7 Cals
- 0 5-a-day

Mustard, English
15g, 1 tbsp

- 1g Protein
- 1g Fat
- 0g Fibre
- 1g Carbs
- 21 Cals
- 0 5-a-day

Mustard, Wholegrain
5g, 1 tsp

- 0g Protein
- 1g Fat
- 0g Fibre
- 0g Carbs
- 7 Cals
- 0 5-a-day

Mustard, Wholegrain
15g, 1 tbsp

- 1g Protein
- 2g Fat
- 1g Fibre
- 1g Carbs
- 21 Cals
- 0 5-a-day

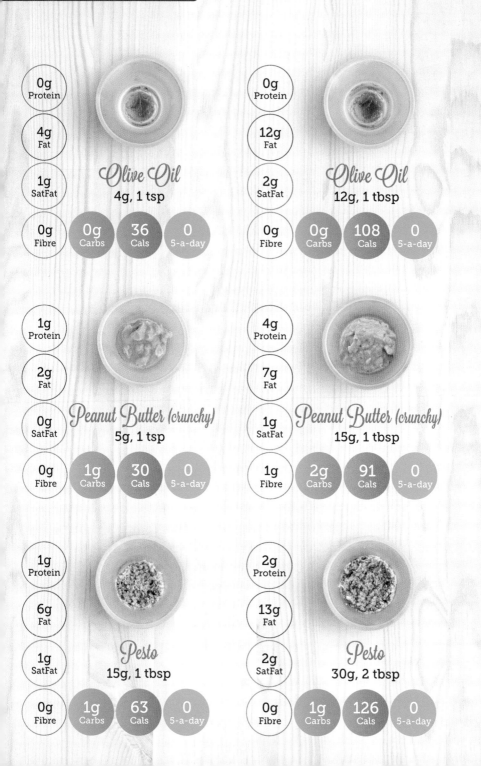

0g
Protein

4g
Fat

1g
SatFat

0g
Fibre

Olive Oil
4g, 1 tsp

0g
Carbs

36
Cals

0
5-a-day

0g
Protein

12g
Fat

2g
SatFat

0g
Fibre

Olive Oil
12g, 1 tbsp

0g
Carbs

108
Cals

0
5-a-day

1g
Protein

2g
Fat

0g
SatFat

0g
Fibre

Peanut Butter (crunchy)
5g, 1 tsp

1g
Carbs

30
Cals

0
5-a-day

4g
Protein

7g
Fat

1g
SatFat

1g
Fibre

Peanut Butter (crunchy)
15g, 1 tbsp

2g
Carbs

91
Cals

0
5-a-day

1g
Protein

6g
Fat

1g
SatFat

0g
Fibre

Pesto
15g, 1 tbsp

1g
Carbs

63
Cals

0
5-a-day

2g
Protein

13g
Fat

2g
SatFat

0g
Fibre

Pesto
30g, 2 tbsp

1g
Carbs

126
Cals

0
5-a-day

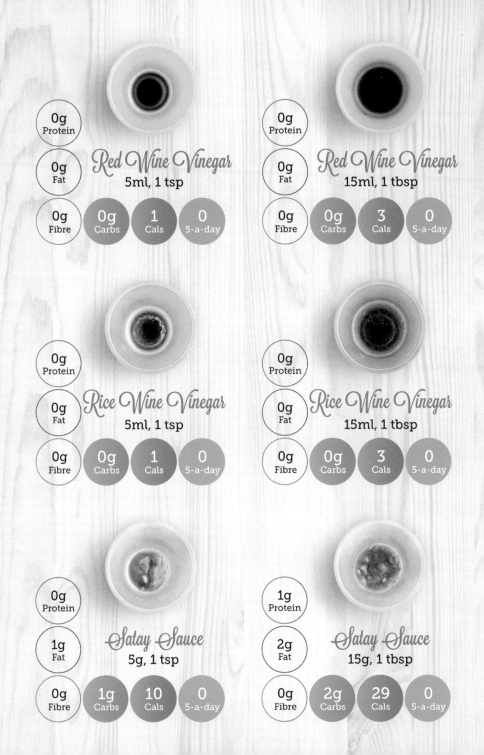

Red Wine Vinegar
5ml, 1 tsp

0g Protein
0g Fat
0g Fibre
0g Carbs
1 Cals
0 5-a-day

Red Wine Vinegar
15ml, 1 tbsp

0g Protein
0g Fat
0g Fibre
0g Carbs
3 Cals
0 5-a-day

Rice Wine Vinegar
5ml, 1 tsp

0g Protein
0g Fat
0g Fibre
0g Carbs
1 Cals
0 5-a-day

Rice Wine Vinegar
15ml, 1 tbsp

0g Protein
0g Fat
0g Fibre
0g Carbs
3 Cals
0 5-a-day

Satay Sauce
5g, 1 tsp

0g Protein
1g Fat
0g Fibre
1g Carbs
10 Cals
0 5-a-day

Satay Sauce
15g, 1 tbsp

1g Protein
2g Fat
0g Fibre
2g Carbs
29 Cals
0 5-a-day

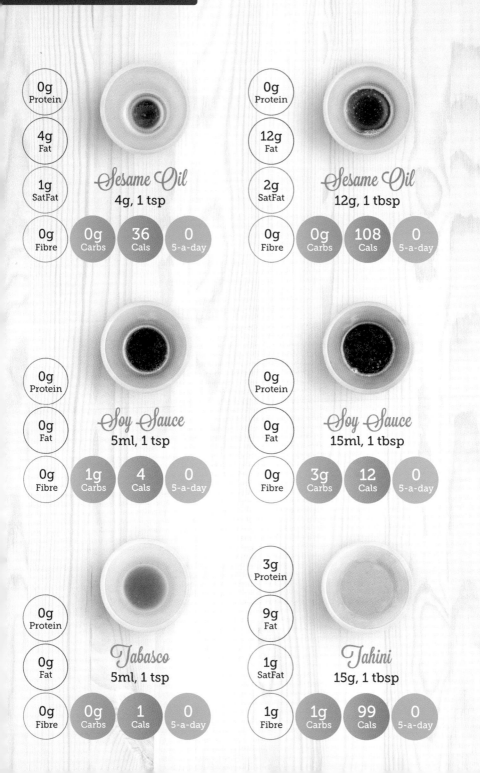

0g Protein
4g Fat
1g SatFat
0g Fibre

Sesame Oil
4g, 1 tsp

0g Carbs
36 Cals
0 5-a-day

0g Protein
12g Fat
2g SatFat
0g Fibre

Sesame Oil
12g, 1 tbsp

0g Carbs
108 Cals
0 5-a-day

0g Protein
0g Fat
0g Fibre

Soy Sauce
5ml, 1 tsp

1g Carbs
4 Cals
0 5-a-day

0g Protein
0g Fat
0g Fibre

Soy Sauce
15ml, 1 tbsp

3g Carbs
12 Cals
0 5-a-day

0g Protein
0g Fat
0g Fibre

Tabasco
5ml, 1 tsp

0g Carbs
1 Cals
0 5-a-day

3g Protein
9g Fat
1g SatFat
1g Fibre

Tahini
15g, 1 tbsp

1g Carbs
99 Cals
0 5-a-day

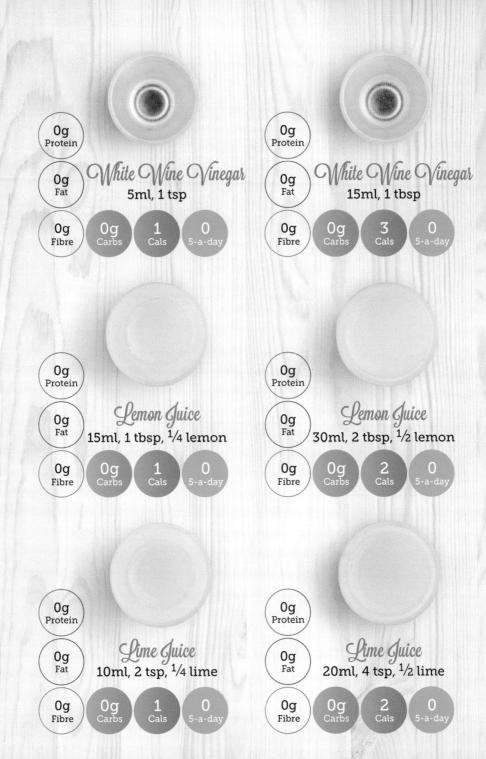

White Wine Vinegar
5ml, 1 tsp

0g Protein
0g Fat
0g Fibre
0g Carbs
1 Cals
0 5-a-day

White Wine Vinegar
15ml, 1 tbsp

0g Protein
0g Fat
0g Fibre
0g Carbs
3 Cals
0 5-a-day

Lemon Juice
15ml, 1 tbsp, ¼ lemon

0g Protein
0g Fat
0g Fibre
0g Carbs
1 Cals
0 5-a-day

Lemon Juice
30ml, 2 tbsp, ½ lemon

0g Protein
0g Fat
0g Fibre
0g Carbs
2 Cals
0 5-a-day

Lime Juice
10ml, 2 tsp, ¼ lime

0g Protein
0g Fat
0g Fibre
0g Carbs
1 Cals
0 5-a-day

Lime Juice
20ml, 4 tsp, ½ lime

0g Protein
0g Fat
0g Fibre
0g Carbs
2 Cals
0 5-a-day

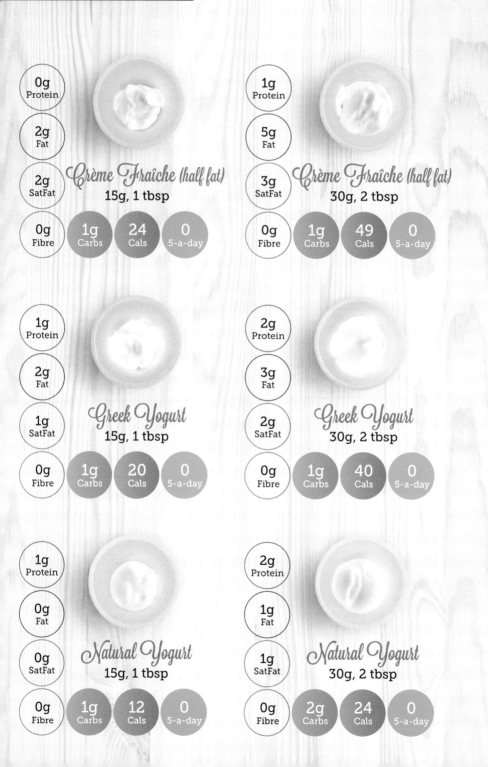

0g Protein
2g Fat
2g SatFat
0g Fibre

Crème Fraîche (half fat)
15g, 1 tbsp

1g Carbs | 24 Cals | 0 5-a-day

1g Protein
5g Fat
3g SatFat
0g Fibre

Crème Fraîche (half fat)
30g, 2 tbsp

1g Carbs | 49 Cals | 0 5-a-day

1g Protein
2g Fat
1g SatFat
0g Fibre

Greek Yogurt
15g, 1 tbsp

1g Carbs | 20 Cals | 0 5-a-day

2g Protein
3g Fat
2g SatFat
0g Fibre

Greek Yogurt
30g, 2 tbsp

1g Carbs | 40 Cals | 0 5-a-day

1g Protein
0g Fat
0g SatFat
0g Fibre

Natural Yogurt
15g, 1 tbsp

1g Carbs | 12 Cals | 0 5-a-day

2g Protein
1g Fat
1g SatFat
0g Fibre

Natural Yogurt
30g, 2 tbsp

2g Carbs | 24 Cals | 0 5-a-day

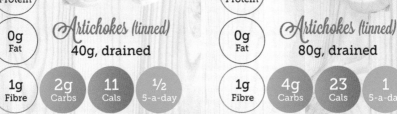

1g Protein

0g Fat

1g Fibre

Asparagus Tips
40g

1g Carbs | **10** Cals | **½** 5-a-day

2g Protein

0g Fat

2g Fibre

Asparagus Tips
80g

2g Carbs | **20** Cals | **1** 5-a-day

1g Protein

0g Fat

0g Fibre

Alfalfa Sprouts
20g

0g Carbs | **5** Cals | **0** 5-a-day

2g Protein

0g Fat

1g Fibre

Alfalfa Sprouts
40g

0g Carbs | **10** Cals | **½** 5-a-day

1g Protein

0g Fat

1g Fibre

Artichokes (tinned)
40g, drained

2g Carbs | **11** Cals | **½** 5-a-day

1g Protein

0g Fat

1g Fibre

Artichokes (tinned)
80g, drained

4g Carbs | **23** Cals | **1** 5-a-day

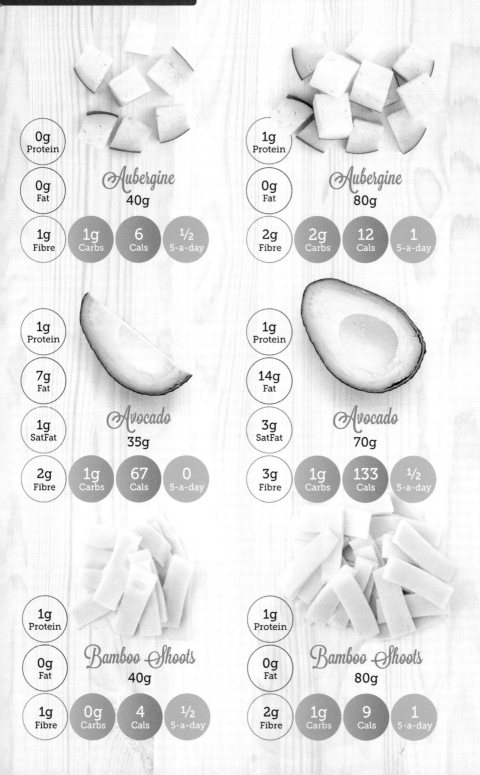

0g Protein

0g Fat

1g Fibre

Aubergine
40g

1g Carbs

6 Cals

½ 5-a-day

1g Protein

0g Fat

2g Fibre

Aubergine
80g

2g Carbs

12 Cals

1 5-a-day

1g Protein

7g Fat

1g SatFat

2g Fibre

Avocado
35g

1g Carbs

67 Cals

0 5-a-day

1g Protein

14g Fat

3g SatFat

3g Fibre

Avocado
70g

1g Carbs

133 Cals

½ 5-a-day

1g Protein

0g Fat

1g Fibre

Bamboo Shoots
40g

0g Carbs

4 Cals

½ 5-a-day

1g Protein

0g Fat

2g Fibre

Bamboo Shoots
80g

1g Carbs

9 Cals

1 5-a-day

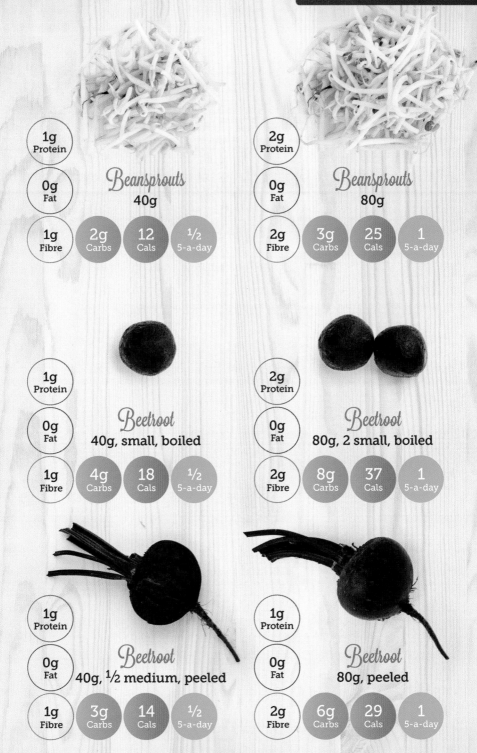

1g Protein

0g Fat

Beansprouts
40g

1g Fibre

2g Carbs

12 Cals

½ 5-a-day

2g Protein

0g Fat

Beansprouts
80g

2g Fibre

3g Carbs

25 Cals

1 5-a-day

1g Protein

0g Fat

Beetroot
40g, small, boiled

1g Fibre

4g Carbs

18 Cals

½ 5-a-day

2g Protein

0g Fat

Beetroot
80g, 2 small, boiled

2g Fibre

8g Carbs

37 Cals

1 5-a-day

1g Protein

0g Fat

Beetroot
40g, ½ medium, peeled

1g Fibre

3g Carbs

14 Cals

½ 5-a-day

1g Protein

0g Fat

Beetroot
80g, peeled

2g Fibre

6g Carbs

29 Cals

1 5-a-day

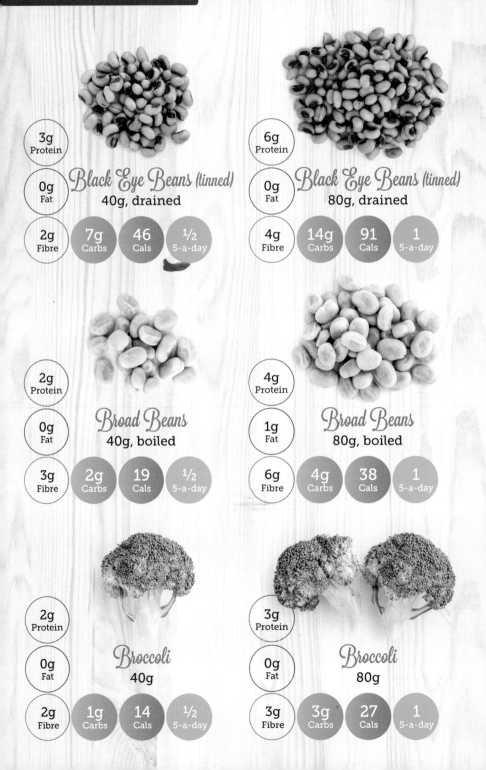

3g Protein

0g Fat

2g Fibre

Black Eye Beans (tinned)
40g, drained

7g Carbs

46 Cals

½ 5-a-day

6g Protein

0g Fat

4g Fibre

Black Eye Beans (tinned)
80g, drained

14g Carbs

91 Cals

1 5-a-day

2g Protein

0g Fat

3g Fibre

Broad Beans
40g, boiled

2g Carbs

19 Cals

½ 5-a-day

4g Protein

1g Fat

6g Fibre

Broad Beans
80g, boiled

4g Carbs

38 Cals

1 5-a-day

2g Protein

0g Fat

2g Fibre

Broccoli
40g

1g Carbs

14 Cals

½ 5-a-day

3g Protein

0g Fat

3g Fibre

Broccoli
80g

3g Carbs

27 Cals

1 5-a-day

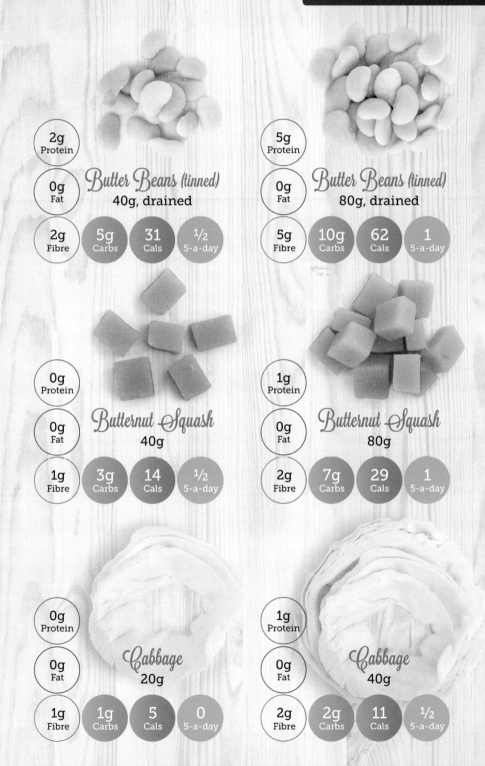

2g Protein

0g Fat

Butter Beans (tinned)
40g, drained

2g Fibre | **5g** Carbs | **31** Cals | **½** 5-a-day

5g Protein

0g Fat

Butter Beans (tinned)
80g, drained

5g Fibre | **10g** Carbs | **62** Cals | **1** 5-a-day

0g Protein

0g Fat

Butternut Squash
40g

1g Fibre | **3g** Carbs | **14** Cals | **½** 5-a-day

1g Protein

0g Fat

Butternut Squash
80g

2g Fibre | **7g** Carbs | **29** Cals | **1** 5-a-day

0g Protein

0g Fat

Cabbage
20g

1g Fibre | **1g** Carbs | **5** Cals | **0** 5-a-day

1g Protein

0g Fat

Cabbage
40g

2g Fibre | **2g** Carbs | **11** Cals | **½** 5-a-day

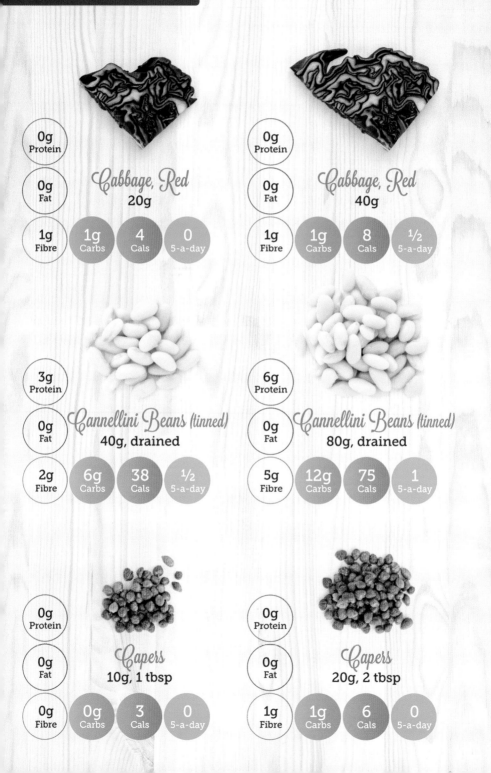

Cabbage, Red
20g

| 0g Protein | 0g Fat | 1g Fibre | 1g Carbs | 4 Cals | 0 5-a-day |

Cabbage, Red
40g

| 0g Protein | 0g Fat | 1g Fibre | 1g Carbs | 8 Cals | ½ 5-a-day |

Cannellini Beans (tinned)
40g, drained

| 3g Protein | 0g Fat | 2g Fibre | 6g Carbs | 38 Cals | ½ 5-a-day |

Cannellini Beans (tinned)
80g, drained

| 6g Protein | 0g Fat | 5g Fibre | 12g Carbs | 75 Cals | 1 5-a-day |

Capers
10g, 1 tbsp

| 0g Protein | 0g Fat | 0g Fibre | 0g Carbs | 3 Cals | 0 5-a-day |

Capers
20g, 2 tbsp

| 0g Protein | 0g Fat | 1g Fibre | 1g Carbs | 6 Cals | 0 5-a-day |

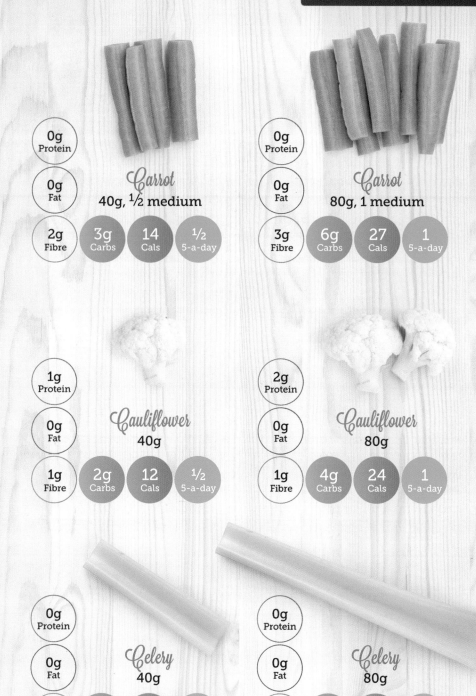

0g Protein

0g Fat

2g Fibre

Carrot
40g, ½ medium

3g Carbs   **14** Cals   **½** 5-a-day

0g Protein

0g Fat

3g Fibre

Carrot
80g, 1 medium

6g Carbs   **27** Cals   **1** 5-a-day

1g Protein

0g Fat

1g Fibre

Cauliflower
40g

2g Carbs   **12** Cals   **½** 5-a-day

2g Protein

0g Fat

1g Fibre

Cauliflower
80g

4g Carbs   **24** Cals   **1** 5-a-day

0g Protein

0g Fat

1g Fibre

Celery
40g

0g Carbs   **3** Cals   **½** 5-a-day

0g Protein

0g Fat

1g Fibre

Celery
80g

1g Carbs   **6** Cals   **1** 5-a-day

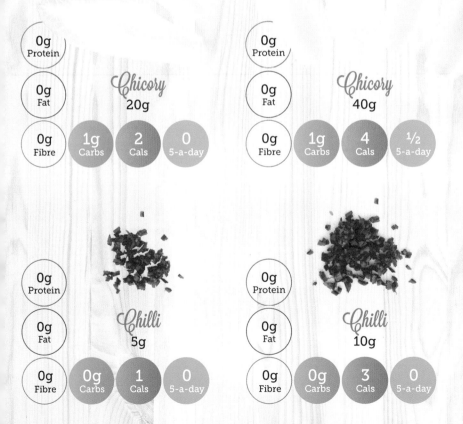

3g Protein

1g Fat

2g Fibre

Chickpeas (tinned)
40g, drained

6g Carbs

46 Cals

½ 5-a-day

6g Protein

2g Fat

4g Fibre

Chickpeas (tinned)
80g, drained

13g Carbs

92 Cals

1 5-a-day

0g Protein

0g Fat

0g Fibre

Chicory
20g

1g Carbs

2 Cals

0 5-a-day

0g Protein

0g Fat

0g Fibre

Chicory
40g

1g Carbs

4 Cals

½ 5-a-day

0g Protein

0g Fat

0g Fibre

Chilli
5g

0g Carbs

1 Cals

0 5-a-day

0g Protein

0g Fat

0g Fibre

Chilli
10g

0g Carbs

3 Cals

0 5-a-day

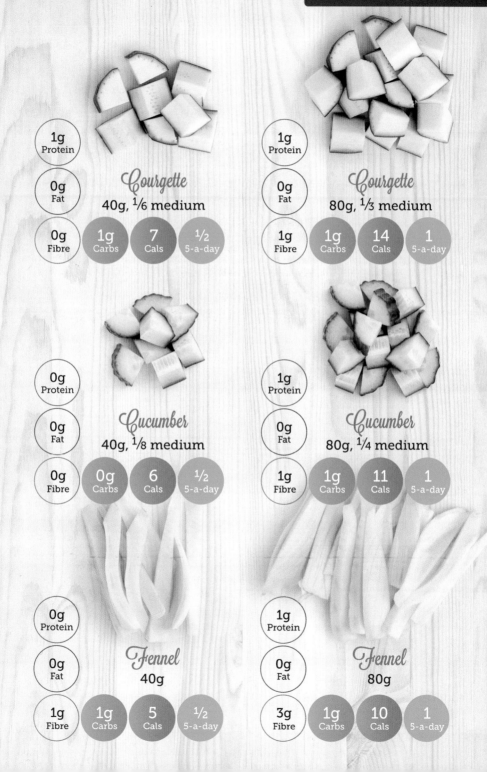

Courgette
40g, ⅙ medium

1g Protein
0g Fat
0g Fibre
1g Carbs
7 Cals
½ 5-a-day

Courgette
80g, ⅓ medium

1g Protein
0g Fat
1g Fibre
1g Carbs
14 Cals
1 5-a-day

Cucumber
40g, ⅛ medium

0g Protein
0g Fat
0g Fibre
0g Carbs
6 Cals
½ 5-a-day

Cucumber
80g, ¼ medium

1g Protein
0g Fat
1g Fibre
1g Carbs
11 Cals
1 5-a-day

Fennel
40g

0g Protein
0g Fat
1g Fibre
1g Carbs
5 Cals
½ 5-a-day

Fennel
80g

1g Protein
0g Fat
3g Fibre
1g Carbs
10 Cals
1 5-a-day

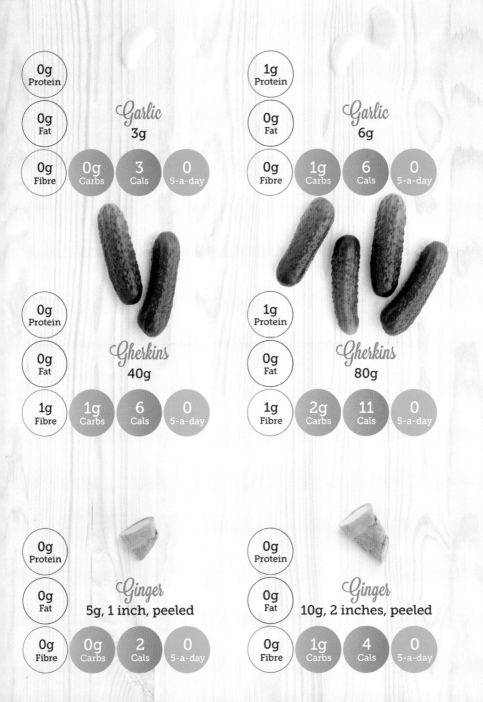

Garlic
3g

0g Protein		
0g Fat		
0g Fibre	0g Carbs	3 Cals	0 5-a-day

Garlic
6g

1g Protein		
0g Fat		
0g Fibre	1g Carbs	6 Cals	0 5-a-day

Gherkins
40g

0g Protein		
0g Fat		
1g Fibre	1g Carbs	6 Cals	0 5-a-day

Gherkins
80g

1g Protein		
0g Fat		
1g Fibre	2g Carbs	11 Cals	0 5-a-day

Ginger
5g, 1 inch, peeled

0g Protein		
0g Fat		
0g Fibre	0g Carbs	2 Cals	0 5-a-day

Ginger
10g, 2 inches, peeled

0g Protein		
0g Fat		
0g Fibre	1g Carbs	4 Cals	0 5-a-day

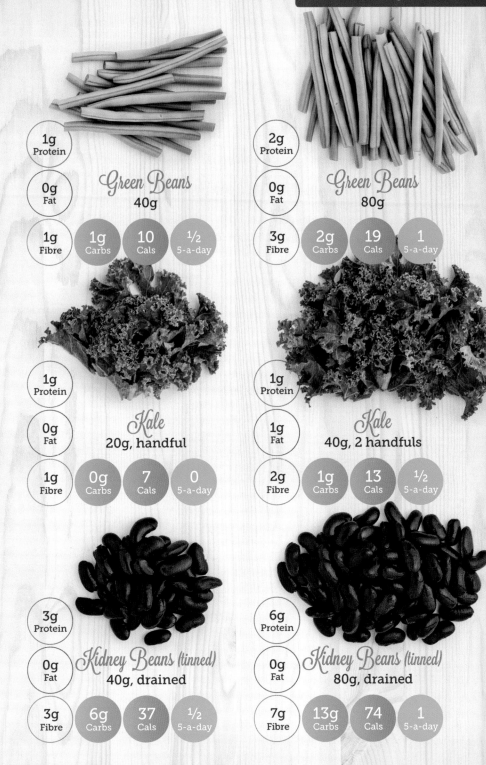

1g Protein

0g Fat

1g Fibre

Green Beans
40g

1g Carbs

10 Cals

½ 5-a-day

2g Protein

0g Fat

3g Fibre

Green Beans
80g

2g Carbs

19 Cals

1 5-a-day

1g Protein

0g Fat

1g Fibre

Kale
20g, handful

0g Carbs

7 Cals

0 5-a-day

1g Protein

1g Fat

2g Fibre

Kale
40g, 2 handfuls

1g Carbs

13 Cals

½ 5-a-day

3g Protein

0g Fat

3g Fibre

Kidney Beans (tinned)
40g, drained

6g Carbs

37 Cals

½ 5-a-day

6g Protein

0g Fat

7g Fibre

Kidney Beans (tinned)
80g, drained

13g Carbs

74 Cals

1 5-a-day

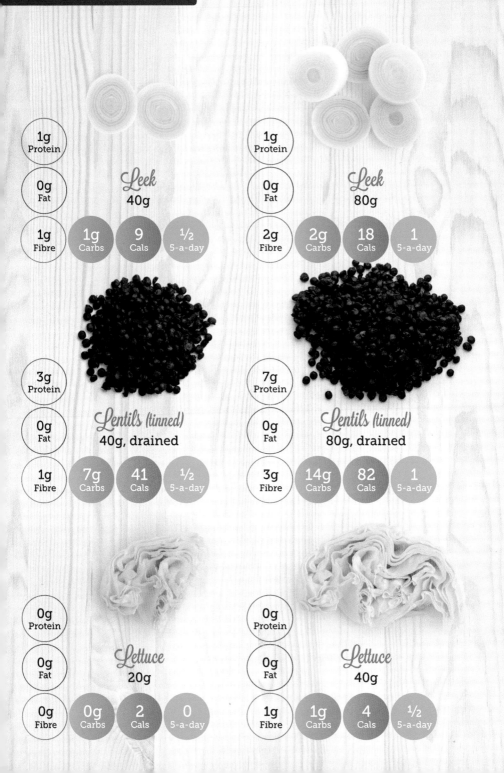

1g Protein
0g Fat
1g Fibre

Leek
40g

1g Carbs | 9 Cals | ½ 5-a-day

1g Protein
0g Fat
2g Fibre

Leek
80g

2g Carbs | 18 Cals | 1 5-a-day

3g Protein
0g Fat
1g Fibre

Lentils (tinned)
40g, drained

7g Carbs | 41 Cals | ½ 5-a-day

7g Protein
0g Fat
3g Fibre

Lentils (tinned)
80g, drained

14g Carbs | 82 Cals | 1 5-a-day

0g Protein
0g Fat
0g Fibre

Lettuce
20g

0g Carbs | 2 Cals | 0 5-a-day

0g Protein
0g Fat
1g Fibre

Lettuce
40g

1g Carbs | 4 Cals | ½ 5-a-day

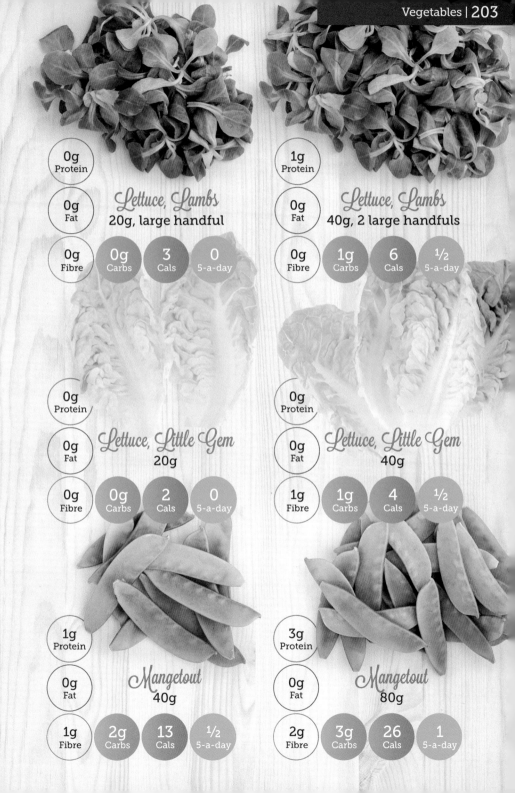

0g Protein

0g Fat

0g Fibre

Lettuce, Lambs
20g, large handful

0g Carbs | **3** Cals | **0** 5-a-day

1g Protein

0g Fat

0g Fibre

Lettuce, Lambs
40g, 2 large handfuls

1g Carbs | **6** Cals | **½** 5-a-day

0g Protein

0g Fat

0g Fibre

Lettuce, Little Gem
20g

0g Carbs | **2** Cals | **0** 5-a-day

0g Protein

0g Fat

1g Fibre

Lettuce, Little Gem
40g

1g Carbs | **4** Cals | **½** 5-a-day

1g Protein

0g Fat

1g Fibre

Mangetout
40g

2g Carbs | **13** Cals | **½** 5-a-day

3g Protein

0g Fat

2g Fibre

Mangetout
80g

3g Carbs | **26** Cals | **1** 5-a-day

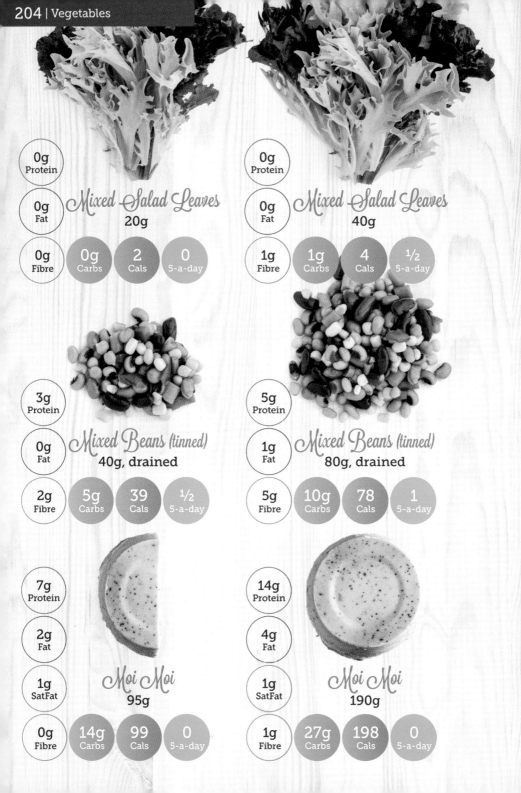

Mixed Salad Leaves
20g

0g Protein
0g Fat
0g Fibre
0g Carbs
2 Cals
0 5-a-day

Mixed Salad Leaves
40g

0g Protein
0g Fat
1g Fibre
1g Carbs
4 Cals
½ 5-a-day

Mixed Beans (tinned)
40g, drained

3g Protein
0g Fat
2g Fibre
5g Carbs
39 Cals
½ 5-a-day

Mixed Beans (tinned)
80g, drained

5g Protein
1g Fat
5g Fibre
10g Carbs
78 Cals
1 5-a-day

Moi Moi
95g

7g Protein
2g Fat
1g SatFat
0g Fibre
14g Carbs
99 Cals
0 5-a-day

Moi Moi
190g

14g Protein
4g Fat
1g SatFat
1g Fibre
27g Carbs
198 Cals
0 5-a-day

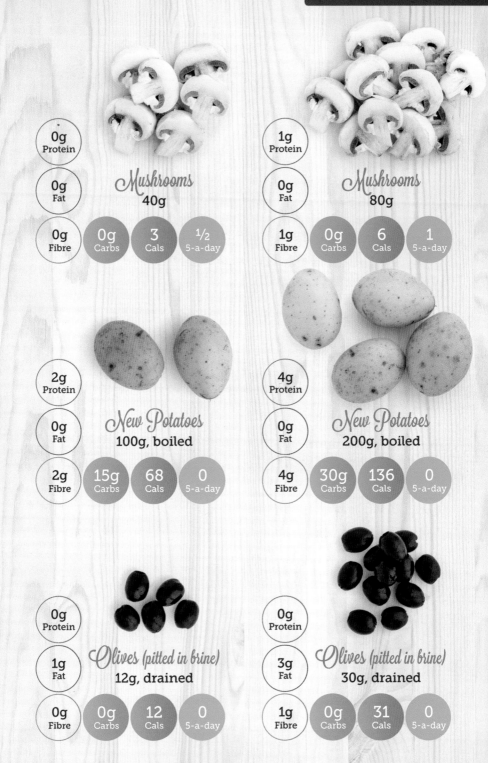

0g
Protein

0g
Fat

0g
Fibre

Mushrooms
40g

0g
Carbs

3
Cals

1/2
5-a-day

1g
Protein

0g
Fat

1g
Fibre

Mushrooms
80g

0g
Carbs

6
Cals

1
5-a-day

2g
Protein

0g
Fat

2g
Fibre

New Potatoes
100g, boiled

15g
Carbs

68
Cals

0
5-a-day

4g
Protein

0g
Fat

4g
Fibre

New Potatoes
200g, boiled

30g
Carbs

136
Cals

0
5-a-day

0g
Protein

1g
Fat

0g
Fibre

Olives (pitted in brine)
12g, drained

0g
Carbs

12
Cals

0
5-a-day

0g
Protein

3g
Fat

1g
Fibre

Olives (pitted in brine)
30g, drained

0g
Carbs

31
Cals

0
5-a-day

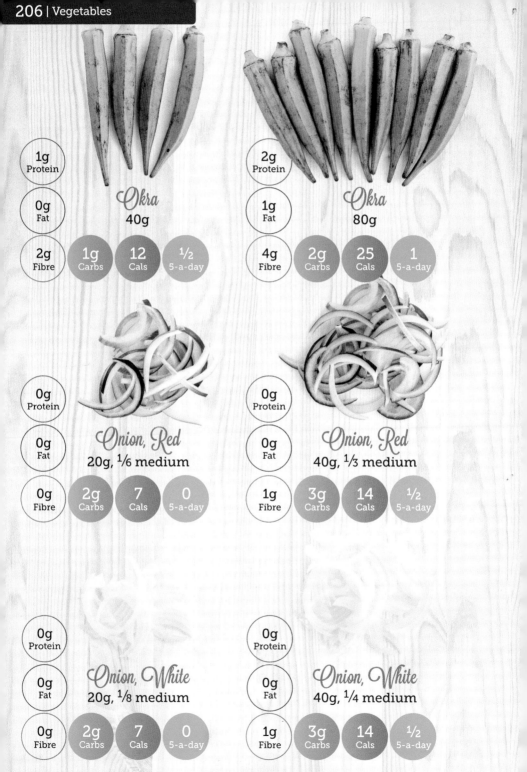

1g
Protein

0g
Fat

2g
Fibre

1g
Carbs

12
Cals

½
5-a-day

Okra
40g

2g
Protein

1g
Fat

4g
Fibre

2g
Carbs

25
Cals

1
5-a-day

Okra
80g

0g
Protein

0g
Fat

0g
Fibre

2g
Carbs

7
Cals

0
5-a-day

Onion, Red
20g, ⅙ medium

0g
Protein

0g
Fat

1g
Fibre

3g
Carbs

14
Cals

½
5-a-day

Onion, Red
40g, ⅓ medium

0g
Protein

0g
Fat

0g
Fibre

2g
Carbs

7
Cals

0
5-a-day

Onion, White
20g, ⅛ medium

0g
Protein

0g
Fat

1g
Fibre

3g
Carbs

14
Cals

½
5-a-day

Onion, White
40g, ¼ medium

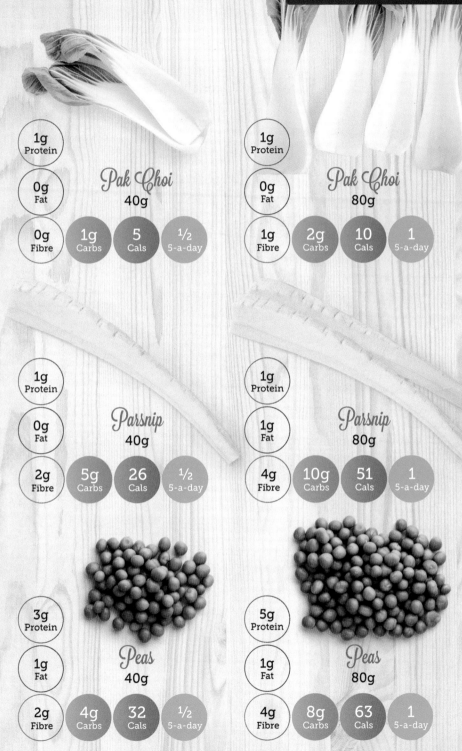

Pak Choi
40g

1g Protein
0g Fat
0g Fibre
1g Carbs
5 Cals
½ 5-a-day

Pak Choi
80g

1g Protein
0g Fat
1g Fibre
2g Carbs
10 Cals
1 5-a-day

Parsnip
40g

1g Protein
0g Fat
2g Fibre
5g Carbs
26 Cals
½ 5-a-day

Parsnip
80g

1g Protein
1g Fat
4g Fibre
10g Carbs
51 Cals
1 5-a-day

Peas
40g

3g Protein
1g Fat
2g Fibre
4g Carbs
32 Cals
½ 5-a-day

Peas
80g

5g Protein
1g Fat
4g Fibre
8g Carbs
63 Cals
1 5-a-day

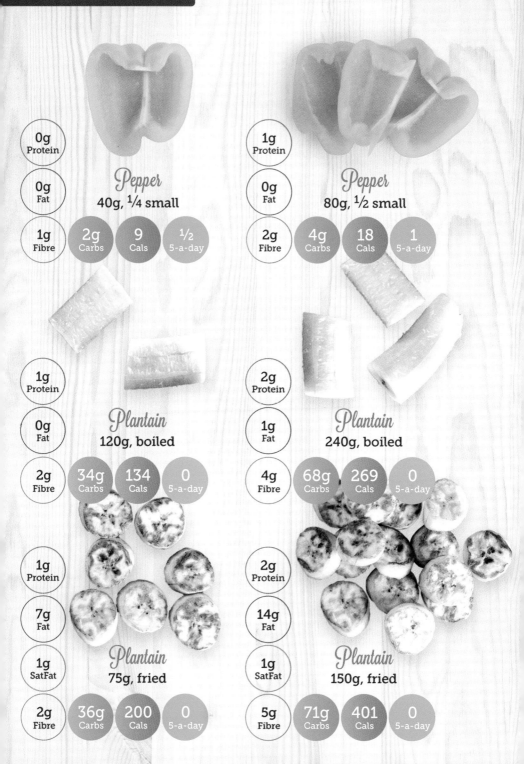

Pepper
40g, ¼ small

Protein	Fat	Fibre	Carbs	Cals	5-a-day
0g	0g	1g	2g	9	½

Pepper
80g, ½ small

Protein	Fat	Fibre	Carbs	Cals	5-a-day
1g	0g	2g	4g	18	1

Plantain
120g, boiled

Protein	Fat	Fibre	Carbs	Cals	5-a-day
1g	0g	2g	34g	134	0

Plantain
240g, boiled

Protein	Fat	Fibre	Carbs	Cals	5-a-day
2g	1g	4g	68g	269	0

Plantain
75g, fried

Protein	Fat	SatFat	Fibre	Carbs	Cals	5-a-day
1g	7g	1g	2g	36g	200	0

Plantain
150g, fried

Protein	Fat	SatFat	Fibre	Carbs	Cals	5-a-day
2g	14g	1g	5g	71g	401	0

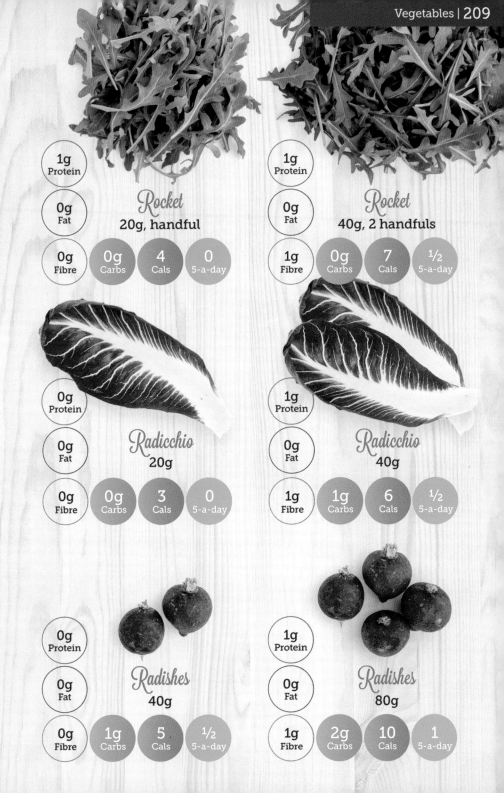

1g Protein

0g Fat

0g Fibre

Rocket
20g, handful

0g Carbs | **4** Cals | **0** 5-a-day

1g Protein

0g Fat

1g Fibre

Rocket
40g, 2 handfuls

0g Carbs | **7** Cals | **½** 5-a-day

0g Protein

0g Fat

0g Fibre

Radicchio
20g

0g Carbs | **3** Cals | **0** 5-a-day

1g Protein

0g Fat

1g Fibre

Radicchio
40g

1g Carbs | **6** Cals | **½** 5-a-day

0g Protein

0g Fat

0g Fibre

Radishes
40g

1g Carbs | **5** Cals | **½** 5-a-day

1g Protein

0g Fat

1g Fibre

Radishes
80g

2g Carbs | **10** Cals | **1** 5-a-day

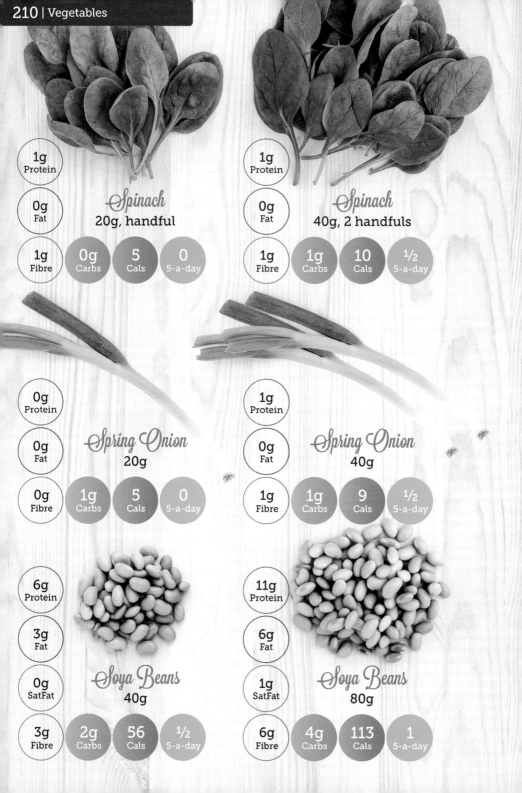

Spinach
20g, handful

- 1g Protein
- 0g Fat
- 1g Fibre
- 0g Carbs
- 5 Cals
- 0 5-a-day

Spinach
40g, 2 handfuls

- 1g Protein
- 0g Fat
- 1g Fibre
- 1g Carbs
- 10 Cals
- ½ 5-a-day

Spring Onion
20g

- 0g Protein
- 0g Fat
- 0g Fibre
- 1g Carbs
- 5 Cals
- 0 5-a-day

Spring Onion
40g

- 1g Protein
- 0g Fat
- 1g Fibre
- 1g Carbs
- 9 Cals
- ½ 5-a-day

Soya Beans
40g

- 6g Protein
- 3g Fat
- 0g SatFat
- 3g Fibre
- 2g Carbs
- 56 Cals
- ½ 5-a-day

Soya Beans
80g

- 11g Protein
- 6g Fat
- 1g SatFat
- 6g Fibre
- 4g Carbs
- 113 Cals
- 1 5-a-day

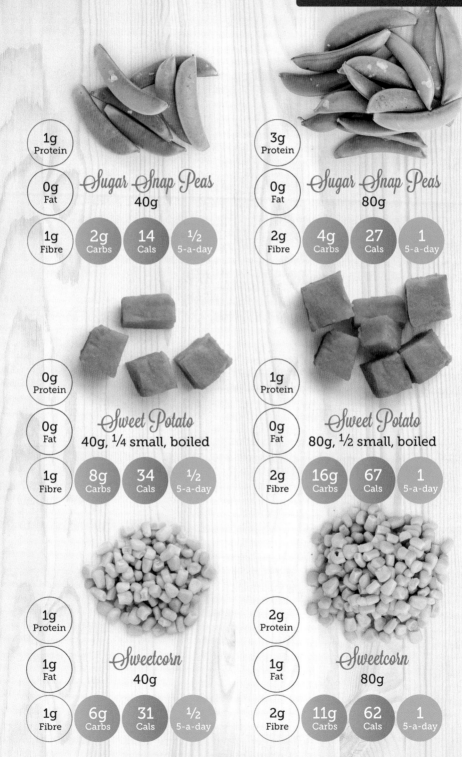

Sugar Snap Peas
40g

1g Protein
0g Fat
1g Fibre
2g Carbs
14 Cals
1/2 5-a-day

Sugar Snap Peas
80g

3g Protein
0g Fat
2g Fibre
4g Carbs
27 Cals
1 5-a-day

Sweet Potato
40g, 1/4 small, boiled

0g Protein
0g Fat
1g Fibre
8g Carbs
34 Cals
1/2 5-a-day

Sweet Potato
80g, 1/2 small, boiled

1g Protein
0g Fat
2g Fibre
16g Carbs
67 Cals
1 5-a-day

Sweetcorn
40g

1g Protein
1g Fat
1g Fibre
6g Carbs
31 Cals
1/2 5-a-day

Sweetcorn
80g

2g Protein
1g Fat
2g Fibre
11g Carbs
62 Cals
1 5-a-day

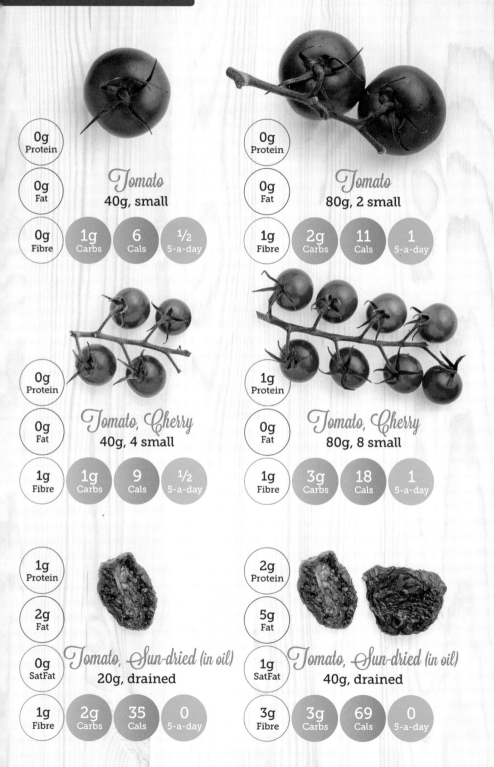

0g Protein
0g Fat
0g Fibre

Tomato
40g, small

1g Carbs | 6 Cals | ½ 5-a-day

0g Protein
0g Fat
1g Fibre

Tomato
80g, 2 small

2g Carbs | 11 Cals | 1 5-a-day

0g Protein
0g Fat
1g Fibre

Tomato, Cherry
40g, 4 small

1g Carbs | 9 Cals | ½ 5-a-day

1g Protein
0g Fat
1g Fibre

Tomato, Cherry
80g, 8 small

3g Carbs | 18 Cals | 1 5-a-day

1g Protein
2g Fat
0g SatFat
1g Fibre

Tomato, Sun-dried (in oil)
20g, drained

2g Carbs | 35 Cals | 0 5-a-day

2g Protein
5g Fat
1g SatFat
3g Fibre

Tomato, Sun-dried (in oil)
40g, drained

3g Carbs | 69 Cals | 0 5-a-day

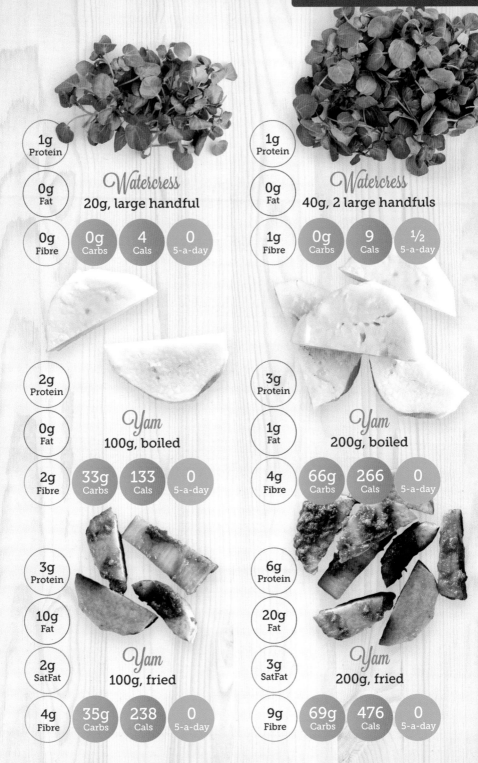

Watercress
20g, large handful

| 1g Protein | 0g Fat | 0g Fibre | 0g Carbs | 4 Cals | 0 5-a-day |

Watercress
40g, 2 large handfuls

| 1g Protein | 0g Fat | 1g Fibre | 0g Carbs | 9 Cals | ½ 5-a-day |

Yam
100g, boiled

| 2g Protein | 0g Fat | 2g Fibre | 33g Carbs | 133 Cals | 0 5-a-day |

Yam
200g, boiled

| 3g Protein | 1g Fat | 4g Fibre | 66g Carbs | 266 Cals | 0 5-a-day |

Yam
100g, fried

| 3g Protein | 10g Fat | 2g SatFat | 4g Fibre | 35g Carbs | 238 Cals | 0 5-a-day |

Yam
200g, fried

| 6g Protein | 20g Fat | 3g SatFat | 9g Fibre | 69g Carbs | 476 Cals | 0 5-a-day |

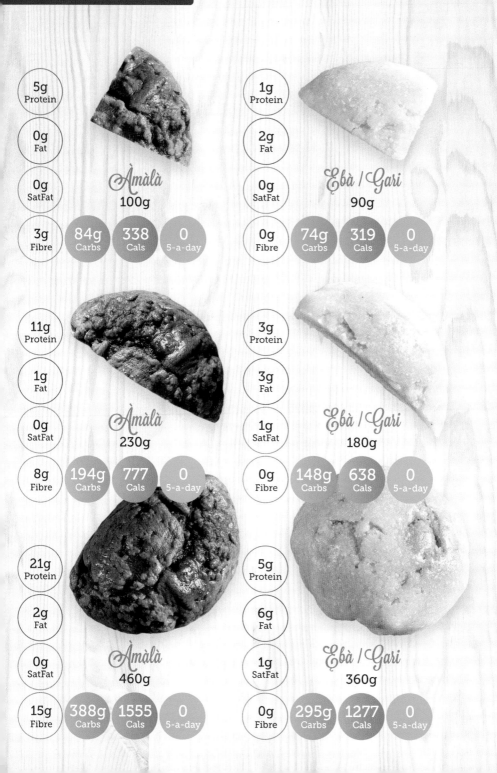

5g Protein
0g Fat
0g SatFat
3g Fibre

Àmàlà
100g

84g Carbs
338 Cals
0 5-a-day

1g Protein
2g Fat
0g SatFat
0g Fibre

Ẹbà / Gari
90g

74g Carbs
319 Cals
0 5-a-day

11g Protein
1g Fat
0g SatFat
8g Fibre

Àmàlà
230g

194g Carbs
777 Cals
0 5-a-day

3g Protein
3g Fat
1g SatFat
0g Fibre

Ẹbà / Gari
180g

148g Carbs
638 Cals
0 5-a-day

21g Protein
2g Fat
0g SatFat
15g Fibre

Àmàlà
460g

388g Carbs
1555 Cals
0 5-a-day

5g Protein
6g Fat
1g SatFat
0g Fibre

Ẹbà / Gari
360g

295g Carbs
1277 Cals
0 5-a-day

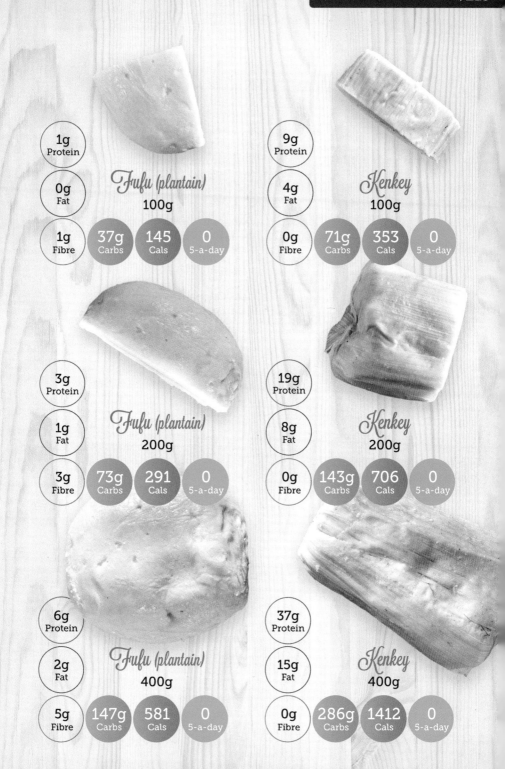

1g Protein

0g Fat

1g Fibre

Fufu (plantain)
100g

37g Carbs

145 Cals

0 5-a-day

9g Protein

4g Fat

0g Fibre

Kenkey
100g

71g Carbs

353 Cals

0 5-a-day

3g Protein

1g Fat

3g Fibre

Fufu (plantain)
200g

73g Carbs

291 Cals

0 5-a-day

19g Protein

8g Fat

0g Fibre

Kenkey
200g

143g Carbs

706 Cals

0 5-a-day

6g Protein

2g Fat

5g Fibre

Fufu (plantain)
400g

147g Carbs

581 Cals

0 5-a-day

37g Protein

15g Fat

0g Fibre

Kenkey
400g

286g Carbs

1412 Cals

0 5-a-day

Recipes

A

Ackee & Saltfish 51, 73
African Bean Stew 53, 124
Asparagus Frittata 90
Avocado & Eggs 42, 64
Avofennel Smoothie 41, 140

B

Baked Aubergine & Feta 85
Beef Lo Mein 48, 101
Beef & Mushroom Stir-fry 89
Beef & Pearl Barley Stew 121
Berries & Jelly 134
Butterbean Dip 51, 138
Butternut Squash Soup 118

C

Carrot & Lentil Soup 46, 125
Cauliflower Risotto 84
Cauli Smoothie 45, 55
Celery & Nut Butter 137
Cheesy Breakfast Mushroom 41, 58
Cheesy Oatcakes 141
Chia Seed Breakfast Pot 44, 62
Chicken & Cashew Stir-fry 40, 102
Chicken Congee Soup 48, 71
Chicken Jollof Rice 105
Chicken, Kale & Chorizo 46, 107
Chicken Tagine 122
Chickpea Patties 94
Chinese Sea Bass 48, 98
Chunky Cottage Pie 99
Classic Cooked Breakfast 59
Coconut Fish Curry 49, 80
Cornmeal Porridge 50, 72

D

Devilled Eggs 138
Dijon Chicken with Mash 41, 106

E

Egg & Mackerel Salad 110
Egg & Quinoa Salad 112

Egg, Salmon & Asparagus 47, 60
Eggs & Fried Plantain 52, 69

F

Fish Pie 42, 103
Fragrant Crab Soup 51, 129
Fruity Porridge 43, 70

G

Groundnut Soup 53, 131
Guacamole 45, 142

J

Jamaican Chicken Curry 50, 79
Jamaican Fish Stew 50, 123
Jerk Chicken 51, 91

K

Kale Crisps 134
Kale Kerfuffle Smoothie 43, 54

L

Lamb Dhansak 76
Lamb & Rosemary Stew 44, 132
Lamb & Spinach Stew 49, 81
Lentil Dal 74

M

Maple Yogurt & Almonds 143
Mexican Chicken Mole 45, 104
Moroccan Veg & Chickpeas 87
Mozzarella & Tomato 142
Mushroom Pepper Omelette 46, 67
Mustard Chicken Salad 109

N

Nigerian Chicken Stew 52, 130

O

Oat Khichdi 49, 66
Okra & Lentil Curry 43, 78
Olive Steak Salad 108

P

Palm Nut Soup 52, 133
Paneer Masala 75
Parsnip Cauliflower Soup 120
Pick up a Pepper Smoothie 47, 140
Pineapple Crispbread 137

Plantain & Beans 97
Pollock & Chickpeas 86
Prawn & Kale Stir-fry 88

Q

Quinoa Stuffed Mushrooms 83

R

Rainbow Tahini Salad 44, **116**
Roasted Pumpkin Seeds 139
Roots & Lentil Salad 40, **117**
Rosemary Olives 135
Rye Bread & Nut Butter 57

S

Salmon Kebabs 45, **100**
Sardines with Salad 53, **65**
Sausage Bean Broth 127
Smoked Salmon & Egg 63
Soya Beans 139
Spiced Broccoli 136
Spicy Chickpeas 143
Spinach Stew & Rice 82
Spring Chicken Soup 42, **128**
Squash & Nut Salad 115
Sweet Potato Curry 77

T

Thai Vegan Salad 113
Tofu & Bean Stir-fry 47, **96**
Tofu Scramble 56
Tuna & Bean Salad 41, **111**
Tuna Lettuce Wraps 53, **141**
Tuna & Roasted Veg 93
Turkey Meatballs 95
Turkey Mushroom Linguine 92
Turkey Rolls 50, **136**
Tuscan Tomato Soup 47, **126**

V

Vanilla Berries 135
Veggie Breakfast 61
Veggie Stew 119

W

Warm Squash Salad 43, **114**

Y

Yogurt, Nuts & Blueberries 40, **68**

Ingredients

A

Ackee 73
Alfalfa Sprouts 108, 116, 191
Almond Butter 137, 182
Almond Milk 62, 172
Almonds 143, 174
Àmàlà 214
Anchovies 152
Apple 54, 55, 70, 115, 156
Apricots 156
    (dried) 122, 166
Artichokes 191
Asafoetida 66
Asparagus 60, 90, 106, 110, 111, 191
Aubergine 78, 85, 87, 93, 119, 192
Avocado 61, 64, 94, 116, 140, 142, 192

B

Baby Corn 142
Bacon 59, 169
Balsamic Vinegar 117, 182
Bamboo Shoots 89, 192
Banana 156
Basil 85, 95, 102, 107, 142, 168
BBQ Sauce 182
Beans
    Black Eye 97, 109, 124, 194
    Broad 194
    Butter 116, 126, 127, 138, 195
    Cannellini 106, 111, 126, 196
    Green 95, 105, 201
    Kidney 79, 201
    Mixed 104, 204
    Soya 115, 139, 210
Beansprouts 88, 89, 101, 113, 193
Beef
    Rump 101
    Sirloin 89, 97, 99, 108, 133, 169
    Stewing 121
    Tomato 142
Beetroot 87, 117, 193
Blackberries 157
Black Eye Beans 97, 109, 124, 194

Blueberries 62, 68, 70, 134, 135, 157
Brazil Nuts 72, 174
Bread 144–145
　Rye 57, 63, 65, 144
Broad Beans 194
Broccoli 102, 106, 112, 116, 128, 132, 136, 194
Bulgur Wheat 85, 179
Butter 75, 80, 183
　Beans 116, 126, 127, 138, 195
Butternut Squash 76, 93, 103, 114, 115, 117, 118, 119, 122, 195

C

Cabbage 98, 99, 105, 113, 127, 128, 129, 132, 195, 196
Cannellini Beans 106, 111, 126, 196
Cantaloupe 157
Capers 196
Cappuccino 150
Carrot 55, 66, 87, 96, 99, 103, 113, 119, 121, 122, 123, 125, 126, 127, 128, 132, 197
Cashews 72, 102, 115, 174
Cauliflower 55, 66, 77, 84, 87, 96, 103, 120, 197
Celery 54, 119, 121, 125, 126, 127, 128, 132, 137, 138, 140, 197
Chana Dal 74
Chapati 145
Cheddar 58, 67, 147
Cheese 58, 67, 83, 84, 85, 92, 103, 106, 107, 117, 137, 141, 142, 147–149
Cherries 158
Cherry Tomato 56, 59, 61, 67, 69, 83, 85, 86, 87, 94, 95, 109, 110, 112, 116, 119, 136, 212
Chestnut Mushrooms 92, 118
Chia Seeds 62, 140
Chicken
　Breast 71, 79, 91, 102, 106, 107, 109, 128, 131, 169
　Drumsticks 130, 170
　Thighs 104, 105, 122
Chickpeas 77, 86, 87, 94, 114, 122, 143, 198
Chicory 198

Chilli 198
　Bean Sauce 96
　Flakes 87, 136, 142
　Oil 129, 183
Chinese Rice Wine 71, 101
Chorizo 107, 170
Coconut 158
　Cream 77
　Milk 80, 129, 172
Cod 80, 152
Coffee 150
Coriander 74, 76, 77, 78, 79, 80, 87, 88, 94, 105, 113, 125, 129, 142, 168
Cornmeal 72
Cottage Cheese 137, 141, 147
Courgette 54, 87, 93, 94, 96, 100, 113, 199
Couscous 180
Crab 129, 152
Cranberries (dried) 166
Crayfish (ground) 124
Cream 103
　Cheese 106, 107
Crème Fraîche 190
Crispbread 137, 144
Cucumber 55, 63, 65, 113, 141, 199

D

Dal 66, 74
Dijon Mustard 100, 106, 117, 138, 185
Dill 60, 63, 100, 103, 108, 111
Dried Fruit 166–167
Dried Shrimp 105, 133
Drinks 150
Drumsticks 130, 170

E

Ebà 214
Edam 147
Egg 59, 60, 61, 63, 64, 67, 69, 90, 94, 95, 110, 112, 138, 151
　Noodles 181
English Mustard 185

F

Fennel 55, 140, 199
Feta 85, 148

Figs 158
   (dried) 166
Fish 73, 86, 98, 100, 103, 110, 111, 123,
   141, 152–155
   Sauce 88, 102, 183
Flour 132
Fruit 156–165
   (dried) 166–167
Fufu 215

G

Galia Melon 159
Garam Masala 74, 80
Gari 214
Garlic 200
Gherkins 200
Ginger 200
Goat's Cheese 117, 148
Goat's Milk 172
Goji Berries 167
Grains 179–180
Grapefruit 159
Grapes 159
Greek Yogurt 62, 84, 110, 115, 125, 190
Green Beans 95, 105, 201

H

Haddock 123
Halloumi 148
Ham 171
Hazelnuts 175
Hemp Milk 172
Herbs 168
Honey 72, 184
Horseradish Sauce 110, 184

I

Icing Sugar 135
Injera 145

J

Jollof Rice 178

K

Kaffir Lime Leaves 129
Kale 54, 87, 88, 97, 107, 114, 126, 134, 201

Kenkey 215
Ketchup 123
Kidney Beans 79, 201
Kiwi 160

L

Lamb 170
   Stewing 76, 81, 132
Lambs Lettuce 203
Latte 150
Leek 119, 126, 202
Lemongrass 102
Lemon Juice 189
Lentils 76, 78, 117, 119, 125, 202
Lettuce 115, 141, 202–203
Lime Juice 189
Linguine 92
Little Gem Lettuce 115, 141, 203
Lychees 160

M

Mackerel 110, 153
Mandarin 160
Mangetout 101, 102, 203
Mango 79, 161
Maple Syrup 62, 143
Mayonnaise 138, 141, 184
Meat 169–171
Melon 157, 159
Milk 70, 172–173
   Almond 62, 172
   Coconut 80, 129, 172
   Goat's 172
   Hemp 172
   Oat 172
   Rice 172
   Soya 72, 173
Mint 87, 102, 116, 138, 168
Moi Moi 204
Mozzarella 142, 149
Muesli 146
Mung Dal 66
Mushrooms 59, 61, 67, 84, 89, 121, 205
   Chestnut 92, 118
   Portobello 58, 83
Mustard 100, 106, 109, 117, 136, 138, 185

N

Natural Yogurt 60, 68, 70, 75, 79, 81, 100, 120, 143, 190
Nectarine 161
Noodles 101, 181
Nuts 68, 70, 72, 102, 115, 174–176

O

Oat Biscuit 146
Oatcake 141, 144
Oat Milk 172
Oats 66, 70, 94, 146
Oil 183, 186, 188
Okra 78, 206
Olive Oil 186
Olives 65, 85, 108, 135, 205
Onion 206
    Spring 71, 101, 102, 112, 113, 116, 123, 129, 141, 210
Orange 161
Oyster Sauce 89, 101

P

Pak Choi 129, 207
Palm Fruit Concentrate 133
Paneer 75
Papaya 162
Paratha 145
Parma Ham 171
Parmesan 84, 92, 103, 149
Parsley 54, 56, 67, 83, 90, 103, 104, 105, 111, 112, 122, 128, 168
Parsnip 106, 117, 120, 121, 207
Passionfruit 162
Pasta 92, 181
Peach 162
Peanut Butter 57, 113, 131, 186
Peanuts 175
Pear 140, 163
Pearl Barley 121, 132, 180
Peas 66, 75, 84, 99, 128, 207
    Sugar Snap 89, 112, 211
Pecans 68, 70, 175
Pepper 56, 58, 65, 66, 67, 69, 73, 75, 78, 79, 87, 88, 89, 93, 97, 100, 101, 104, 107, 113, 114, 116, 119, 123, 129, 131, 140, 208

Persimmon 163
Pesto 186
Petit Pois 75, 84
Pineapple 137, 140, 163
Pine Nuts 176
Pistachios 176
Pitta Bread 145
Plantain 69, 97, 208
Plum 164
Pollock 86, 103, 123
Pomegranate Seeds 115, 164
Pork Sausage 127
Portobello Mushroom 58, 83
Potatoes 99, 205
    Sweet 77, 95, 211
Prawns 88, 103, 153
Pumpkin Seeds 112, 114, 115, 139, 177
Puy Lentils 117

Q

Quinoa 83, 112, 180
Quorn 151

R

Radicchio 209
Radishes 113, 209
Raisins 167
Raspberries 135, 164
Red Leicester 149
Red Wine 132
Red Wine Vinegar 117, 187
Rice 178–179
    Basmati 71, 82, 105
    Milk 172
    Noodles 101
    & Peas 179
    Wine 71, 101
    Wine Vinegar 113, 187
Ricotta 83
Rocket 56, 63, 95, 209
Rosemary 84, 85, 93, 95, 99, 118, 121, 126, 127, 132, 135, 168
Rump Beef 101
Rye Bread 57, 63, 65, 144
Rye Crispbread 137

S

Salad Leaves 109, 110, 116, 204
Salmon 60, 63, 100, 153, 154
Saltfish 73
Sardines 65, 154
Satay Sauce 187
Satsuma 165
Sauces 182–190
Sausage 127, 171
Savoy Cabbage 99
Scallops 155
Sea Bass 98
Seeds 177
Sesame Oil 71, 98, 101, 113, 188
Sesame Seeds 177
Shrimp (dried) 105, 133
Sirloin Beef 89, 97, 99, 108, 133, 169
Smoked Salmon 60, 63, 154
Soya Beans 88, 115, 139, 210
Soya Milk 72, 173
Soy Sauce 71, 88, 89, 91, 96, 98, 101,
    113, 188
Spaghetti 92
Spelt Bread 144
Spinach 59, 61, 76, 81, 82, 86, 94, 103,
    111, 131, 133, 140, 210
Split Lentils 76, 78, 119, 125
Spreads & Sauces 182–190
Spring Onion 71, 101, 102, 112, 113,
    116, 123, 129, 141, 210
Squash 76, 93, 103, 114, 115, 117, 118,
    119, 122, 195
Strawberries 117, 134, 135, 165
Sugar Snap Peas 89, 112, 211
Sultanas 167
Sun-dried Tomato 90, 212
Sunflower Seeds 116, 177
Sweetcorn 211
Sweet Potato 77, 95, 211
Syrup 62, 143

T

Tabasco 138, 188
Tahini 112, 114, 115, 116, 188
Tarragon 106, 109
Tea 150
Thai Basil 102

Thyme 84, 91, 95, 99, 115, 118, 119,
    120, 121, 127, 128, 168
Tofu 56, 96, 113, 151
Tomato 73, 74, 75, 77, 79, 80, 82, 103,
    105, 108, 123, 124, 130, 131, 133,
    142, 212
    Beef 142
    Cherry 56, 59, 61, 67, 69, 83, 85, 86,
        87, 94, 95, 109, 110, 112, 116,
        119, 136, 212
    Ketchup 123
    Purée 73, 105, 130, 132
    Sun-dried 90, 212
    Tinned 76, 104, 121, 122, 126
Trout 155
Tuna 93, 111, 141, 155
Turkey 136
    Breast 92, 171
    Mince 95

V

Vanilla 62, 72, 135
Vegetables 191–213
Vinegar
    Balsamic 117, 182
    Red Wine 117, 187
    Rice Wine 113, 187
    White Wine 109, 111, 189

W

Walnuts 115, 176
Watercress 58, 83, 108, 117, 213
Watermelon 165
Wheat Biscuit 146
Whipping Cream 103
White Wine Vinegar 109, 111, 189
Wholegrain Mustard 109, 136, 185
Wild Rice 179
Worcestershire Sauce 121

Y

Yam 213
Yogurt
    Greek 62, 84, 110, 115, 125, 190
    Natural 60, 68, 70, 75, 79, 81, 100,
        120, 143, 190

About the Authors

Chris Cheyette BSc (Hons) MSc RD
Diabetes Specialist Dietitian

Chris is a Diabetes Specialist Dietitian within the NHS, working with people with type 1, type 2 and gestational diabetes. Chris has spearheaded a number of projects over the years, many with the aim of improving diabetes educational resources. These include an educational DVD for young people with diabetes, which earned him the 2007 British Dietetic Association Elizabeth Washington Award. Chris has also published a number of journal articles on weight management and diabetes. He regularly undertakes local and national presentations to healthcare professionals, has done TV & newspaper interviews, and has participated as a guest expert in online discussions.

Yello Balolia BA (Hons)
Entrepreneur & Creative Photographer

Having achieved a first class honours degree in Photography, Canada-born, Blackpool-bred and now London-based Yello used his entrepreneurial and creative skills to found Chello Publishing Limited with Chris Cheyette, to publish Carbs & Cals (**www.carbsandcals.com**), the bestselling and multi-award-winning book and app for diabetes and weight management. He has also undertaken a series of creative projects including private commissions (**www.yellobalolia.com**), a ukulele book for beginners (**www.ukulology.com**), and most recently a 3-day festival, inspiring people to be their most positive, social and authentic selves (**www.magicalfestival.co.uk**).

Awards

Carbs & Cals won **Best Dietary Management Initiative** at the Quality in Care Awards 2014

The Carbs & Cals App won **New Product of the Year** in the Complete Nutrition Awards 2012

Carbs & Cals won the BDA Dame Barbara Clayton **Award for Innovation & Excellence** 2011

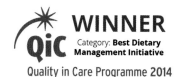

WINNER
Category: **Best Dietary Management Initiative**
Quality in Care Programme 2014

The Association of UK Dietitians
Winner of the 2011 Dame Barbara Clayton Award

Carbs & Cals APP
WINNER
NEW PRODUCT OF THE YEAR

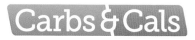

Carbs & Cals

Carbs & Cals APP

Available for iOS & Android

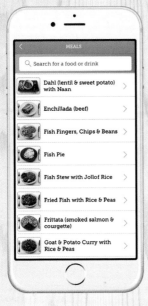

★ Over 3,500 food photos, including branded items

★ Perfect for weight loss, portion control & diabetes

★ The ultimate portable carb & calorie counter!

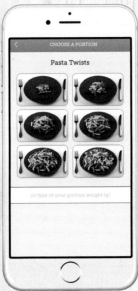

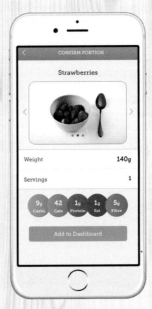

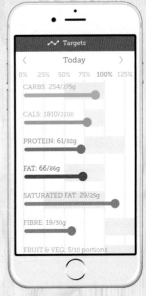

www.carbsandcals.com

MORE FROM Carbs & Cals

Visual resources for diabetes, weight loss & healthy eating

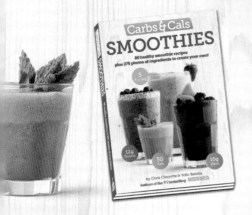

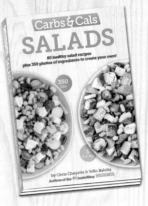

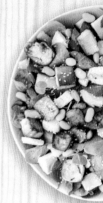

SMOOTHIES

★ 80 delicious smoothie recipes

★ Values for carbs, calories, protein, fat, fibre and 5-a-day fruit & veg

SALADS

★ 80 easy & great-tasting salads

★ Includes low-cal, high-fibre and 5-a-day recipes

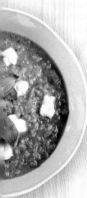

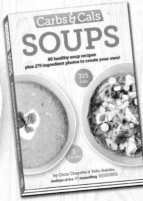

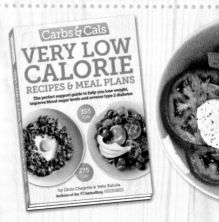

SOUPS

★ 80 quick and tasty single-portion soup recipes

★ Includes 10 mega soups containing all 5 of your 5-a-day!

VERY LOW CALORIE
RECIPES & MEAL PLANS

★ Meal plans to help weight loss

★ Ideal for managing type 2 diabetes and pre-diabetes